"In this very readable text, Koman and Keane share essential lessons they have learned during 40 years of work in behavioral health systems of care. They describe why systems of care are needed, how they can be designed and operated effectively, how they can achieve good person-centered outcomes, and what the future is likely to portend. Excellent case studies and examples are provided at every step on this delightful journey. Students embarking on graduate training in behavioral healthcare will find this text to be very useful, as will system of care managers, clinicians, and consultants seeking to improve care access, quality, and outcome, while controlling cost. A practical text of this type is long overdue in the behavioral healthcare field."

Ron Manderscheid, PhD, *Adjunct Professor, Bloomberg School of Public Health, Johns Hopkins University and Suzanne Dworak Peck School of Social Work, University of Southern California*

"The authors offer a comprehensive evaluation of the history of mental health care and a practical guide to creating a true system of behavioral health care to facilitate excellent treatment and a path to individual healing and recovery. Given the explosion of demand for behavioral health post pandemic, this book could not be timelier."

Marylou Sudders, MSW, ACSW, *Former Commissioner of Mental Health and Secretary of Health and Human Services, Commonwealth of Massachusetts, USA*

"Two dedicated and experienced experts provide a guide in mission driven care while balancing clinical and business concerns. Having accomplished this dance in multiple settings, the authors share best practices to follow, and examples of lessons learned. This book is a must read for entrepreneurs as well as mental health leaders navigating the changing behavioral health landscape."

Kenneth L. Weiner, MD, *Founder of Eating Recovery Center and Pathlight Behavioral*

DESIGNING AND OPERATING A SYSTEM OF CARE IN BEHAVIORAL HEALTH

Designing and Operating a System of Care in Behavioral Health: Solutions to Fragmentation in Mental Health proposes a pathway to combat the current fragmentation of mental health services.

Drawing on the authors' 25 years of experience in the private and public sectors, this book develops a constellation of integrated treatment services to provide a cohesive path to recovery for individuals with mental or behavioral disorders. Koman and Keane embrace the request by patients and their families to be "at the table" in making decisions about their care and to influence how this care is provided by professionals and institutions.

This is an invaluable reference for mental and behavioral health professionals seeking a better way to provide effective mental health services to clients and their families.

Stuart L. Koman is co-founder, former president, and CEO of Walden Behavioral Care. For over 25 years, he has developed innovative behavioral healthcare services and products in private and public sectors with an emphasis on advanced clinical design and sound business planning.

Robert J. Keane is a senior behavioral health administrator with more than 40 years of experience treating diverse patient populations within the mental health system. He is a recognized expert on adolescent eating disorders and the challenges of isolation that teens experience through social media.

DESIGNING AND OPERATING A SYSTEM OF CARE IN BEHAVIORAL HEALTH

Solutions to Fragmentation in Mental Health

Stuart L. Koman and Robert J. Keane

Routledge
Taylor & Francis Group
NEW YORK AND LONDON

Designed cover image: taweesak petphuang © Getty Images

First published 2025
by Routledge
605 Third Avenue, New York, NY 10158

and by Routledge
4 Park Square, Milton Park, Abingdon, Oxon, OX14 4RN

Routledge is an imprint of the Taylor & Francis Group, an informa business

Library of Congress Cataloging-in-Publication Data
Names: Koman, Stuart L., 1954– author. | Keane, Robert J., author.
Title: Designing and operating a system of care in behavioral health : solutions to fragmentation in mental health / Stuart L. Koman, Robert J. Keane.
Description: New York, NY : Routledge, 2025. |
Includes bibliographical references and index. |
Identifiers: LCCN 2024031793 (print) | LCCN 2024031794 (ebook) |
ISBN 9781138038455 (hardback) | ISBN 9781138038462 (paperback) |
ISBN 9781315177366 (ebook)
Subjects: LCSH: Mental health services. | Integrated delivery of health care.
Classification: LCC RA790 .K59 2025 (print) | LCC RA790 (ebook) |
DDC 362.2–dc23/eng/20240816
LC record available at https://lccn.loc.gov/2024031793
LC ebook record available at https://lccn.loc.gov/2024031794

ISBN: 978-1-138-03845-5 (hbk)
ISBN: 978-1-138-03846-2 (pbk)
ISBN: 978-1-315-17736-6 (ebk)

DOI: 10.4324/9781315177366

Typeset in Times New Roman
by Newgen Publishing UK

CONTENTS

ACKNOWLEDGMENTS

Stuart L. Koman

Early in my career, I said that I never wanted to write a book or teach a course unless I had enough real-world experience to make it useful. Forty years later, I'm thinking maybe I over thought this point, but at least I'm still here to write the story. And writing the story requires acknowledging all of the people who helped along the way, a very tall task since this group legitimately encompasses hundreds of colleagues/collaborators and tens of thousands of consumers/patients who allowed me to promote an "us" with three different and unique behavioral healthcare organizations. I wish to thank these participants for their patience and tolerance and more specifically their trust in me to lead them through many years and phases of becoming the healing communities that they ultimately did.

This book would not have happened without the patience, energy, and talent of my co-author, Bob Keane. I am indebted to him for his many contributions to the clinical and business ventures that I started; our paths aligned again and again over a forty-year span making it second nature for us to work together on this project, but it was Bob's foresight and perseverance that got this idea through the pandemic and then into production, and it's been his quiet tenacity and natural ability to turn a phrase that has brought us to completion. My friend for the ages, Dr. Len Rosen, is always my model of literary achievement; I thank him for inspiration, expressions of confidence, and an early read and editorial guidance of the manuscript.

Many others deserve mention as co-conspirators and idea contributors along the way. Maggie Moran, Patricia Sutherland, Gail Hanson-Mayer, Paula Vass, Jim Greenblatt, Ken Minkoff, Chuck Rossignol, Ken Sklar, Richard

Kadison, and Michael Krupa all played major roles at various times. Russ Ricci, David and Len Fassler, Larry Cohen, Walter Henritze, Tom Taylor, Michael Papile, and Jed Donahue were instrumental business associates, starting and/or keeping the enterprises afloat. Bill Mosakowski made contributions in all areas and was steadfast in his support through the ups and downs. Joan Mikula, Marylou Sudders, and Ann Capoccia were early supporters, saw promise in many of the ideas in this book, and put the trust of the Commonwealth of Massachusetts behind them.

Finally, I thank my mentor of all mentors, my father, Bernie Koman who was a singular loving presence to me and an exceptional model as a community and enterprise builder, business consultant and one person safety net. Over the years, we faced the risks together; he survived long enough to revel in the achievements of his son, as did my mother Toby, none of which would have been possible without him. This legacy flows through me to my children, Jason and Candace and Kyra and my grandson, Jack – they have inspired me every day of my life since they arrived.

Robert J. Keane

I feel incredibly fortunate to work in behavioral health. Over the course of my career, I've been able to provide direct care as a clinician, and to work as an administrator, a regulator, a payer, and an educator. My teachers have been the many patients and families that I have had the privilege to know and work with. And at every step of the way I have been profoundly influenced by my colleagues, truly extraordinary people. I am grateful for their dedication, curiosity, and kindness every day.

This book has been informed by the organizations and people I have known and worked with. Undertaking and completing this project has required me to think back over many treatment settings and to consider what has worked (sometimes very well) and what still needs to happen. I am indebted to those programs and institutions, and people within them and deeply appreciate their patience and the tremendous support I have received. You have made my work enriching and enjoyable.

I'd like to thank my wife Sharon, one of the most talented behavioral health professionals I know. She has been my personal consultant and sounding board over these years. Thank you also to our three daughters, Miranda, Aisling, and Rose. As a family, they have tolerated with good humor the time I've spent in my work and the challenges that are part of the job.

And last, I'd like to thank my co-author, Stuart Koman. Stu has been both a friend and mentor since I entered the field. I had the good fortune of meeting him four decades ago and we've worked together through three systems of care. It is his thinking that has crafted these systems of care and informs much of this book. He's a proven leader in behavioral health, capable of balancing the clinical and business demands of an organization while maintaining a clear focus on mission. Most importantly, he has been a consistent support and guide in my life, always pushing me to grow personally and develop professionally. It has been an honor to do this project with him.

The authors especially wish to acknowledge Baila Punch, for her work in managing the manuscript, refining the graphics and keeping us focused, always with kindness and patience.

INTRODUCTION

A Behavioral Health System of Care

Central to our discourse is the concept of a "Behavioral Health System of Care," which we define as a coordinated network of treatment services meticulously designed to holistically address the needs of individuals with serious behavioral health disorders. Unlike conventional fragmented approaches, a Behavioral Health System of Care offers a cohesive and rational path to recovery, encompassing various interventions tailored to the individual's unique circumstances.

As we stand at a pivotal juncture in healthcare evolution, characterized by industry consolidation and post-pandemic uncertainties, *Designing and Operating a System of Care in Behavioral Health: Solutions to Fragmentation in Mental Health* serves as a timely call to action. By leveraging lessons from the past and advocating for a systemic shift toward comprehensive care models, we aspire to catalyze meaningful change and enhance the well-being of individuals and families grappling with mental health challenges.

We feel both obliged and compelled to write this book. The ideas in it have been developed over the course of our careers, and through that time, there have been many forms and approaches to treatment for mental disorders. Many have provided some relief to the users and are worthy of continued development and use; however, we have come to the firm belief that in most respects the field of behavioral health has missed the mark for what our most vulnerable population of users really needs to get well. We are not alone in this conclusion (Insel 2022). In fact, most of the time, behavioral healthcare is disruptive. It is provided in a fragmented, chaotic manner. In reality, we ask people in the midst of episodes of mood and cognitive impairment to navigate their way through

DOI: 10.4324/9781315177366-1

program after program and often start over with a new provider that will most likely have a different expertise and philosophy of treatment than the previous one. Failure is common and frustration is ubiquitous..

The focus of this book is a "system of care," and we believe that it is the antidote to fragmentation and the drastically escalating cost in healthcare. Over the years, the term has been used liberally by behavioral healthcare marketers along with the term "continuum" to describe a grouping of programs or services that relate to a specific age, diagnostic category, or geographic area. Unfortunately, the term is often used improperly; there is nothing "systemic" about the programs being described, and more often, the programs in the system function independently with little or no connection to any other program. We use the term "system of care" and Behavioral Health System of Care (BHSoC) quite specifically to refer to a "constellation of treatment services intentionally developed to work together in a coordinated manner to provide a cohesive and rational path to recovery for individuals with a particular serious mental or behavioral disorder." This definition has many implications, and we will break it down into its component parts and review each part in detail as we work our way through this book.

The concept of a system of care has been around for some time. It was a particularly active terminology in the 1990s and seems to have fallen off the radar to a large extent after 2005 or so. Without question, we were influenced by those people and agencies that were concerned about child welfare and child and adolescent behavioral health (Knitzer 1982; Stroul and Friedman 1986). They reasoned, quite rightly, that a child in the throes of a serious mental or behavioral disorder was subject to an array of influences from family and community that all had to be understood and addressed for the child to get better (Behar 1986; Friesen and Koroloff 1990). Appreciating the importance of family and community systems on an individual child or adolescent led to a broadening of thinking about how to therapeutically create an impact by using multiple services and points of intervention. The term "wraparound" was coined to describe "wrapping services around the child and family," creating a broader lens through which to view diverse services like housing support, home-based parental skills training, and therapeutic summer camp along with individual and family therapy, psychopharmacology, and hospital or residential treatment when necessary.

Other major influences, especially the advent and initial implementation of "managed care" appeared around the same time. The central idea driving the emergence of managed care was the belief on the part of employers that treatment costs were out of control. Communicated to their insurers was the need for containment and, as importantly, that cost was unrelated to positive outcome. In other words, behavioral health providers were spending a lot of money with no or limited appreciable benefit to those being treated.

This began as early as the 1980s when private psychiatric hospitals emerged as an alternative to an overcrowded and troubled state hospital system. Rather than being paid for by tax dollars (as was the state system), private psychiatric hospitals were paid by insurance companies from a covered benefit. Private psychiatric hospitals grew, along with a growing awareness of the role that medication could play in making a troubled person well. Hospitals expanded as did the numbers of individuals they treated. In fact, they grew faster than any other part of the healthcare system (Broskowski 1991).

Administrators in these hospitals developed their own admission procedures and hours (often limited to business hours) and carefully screened who would be admitted. Left unchecked, the time a person stayed in a facility, the "length of stay" was predictably lengthy. In fact, lengths of stay were so long that the best indicator of length of stay in a private psychiatric hospital turned out to be equal to the covered benefit in a person's insurance coverage. That meant that the more liberal your insurance policy benefit (and at that time, most were quite generous), the longer your length of stay. The disorder being treated and even the severity of your symptoms did not seem to matter (Fisher et al. 2001).

In many respects, the private insurance industry had been caught off guard and was unprepared for the expansive growth. For a number of years, all they could do was pay claims, which unintentionally gave license to more growth. Soon, payers became more sophisticated in tracking how their money was being spent. The extravagance of behavioral health became a clear and easy target. Cost containment in behavioral health developed in part through the demands of businesses that purchased health insurance and their need to reduce costs that had been passed onto their employees. Managed care was born and the scrutiny that befell the behavioral health industry changed it forever.

A third major influence that took root during this time is clearly the demand by consumers and families to be "at the table" in making decisions about their care. For the first time, consumers were coming out of the shadows of stigma and fear to speak on their own behalf and try to influence the way that governments and insurers spend money on care and shape the way that professionals and institutions provide the care (Fisher 1994; Sluyter 1994; Salzer 1997). It is pretty clear that this movement will sustain and grow and ultimately be the strongest influence on healthcare in this century.

All of this is to say that we come about our work in systems of care honestly. We are two senior level clinicians and administrators who, remarkably, have worked together over thirty years and through three distinct systems of care. Through that time, we have learned that systems of care are challenging; they're hard to build and require vigilance to keep them true to their intended focus. And despite their current imperfections and all the work they require, we firmly believe that in behavioral health, systems of care are essential. They offer the best chance for a positive treatment experience for a patient and their family. We also believe that a system of care is one of the most viable business models in a field that over decades has struggled to make ends meet. A well running system of care provides a consistent customer base, a quality product, and expanding referrals.

Yet, truth be told, while many behavioral health organizations today will profess to have a working system of care, and most will make remarkable claims of their effectiveness, in our experience, most systems of care fail to meet both their professed clinical outcomes and lofty business goals. Additionally, many of the behavioral health professionals employed in these systems are ill equipped, and at times resistant to making a behavioral health system work as an integrated system. For most, systems of care are not intuitive, and arguably, systems are counter to the training and orientation that most behavioral health clinicians are familiar with. As a group, we are trained and grow into practitioners who work in private, often focused on one patient at a time in one treatment setting. What happens in our office with a patient or family is rarely shared and we have little investment in making a transition to another level of care, especially if the patient has good health insurance or the ability to pay privately. We have learned to resist sharing our clinical experiences as some may be judged harshly if the client is not "cured" or doing much better. Lack of success with a patient is perceived as a weakness or lack of talent and maybe even as clinical failure. In these cases, it is often easier to blindly pass off a difficult client or family to another setting or practitioner where the blame for lack of progress rests with either the patient or colleague.

And for many patients, the current practice works well or well enough. Most individuals present with problems that while not minimal do not present a high degree of risk and they respond well to once a week individual therapy or lower level intervention. However, what works for this population is woefully inadequate for individuals who are struggling with a severe and persistent mental illness. A different level of service is required, and, in order for treatment to truly be effective, it has to occur in a system.

In a functioning system of care, blaming the patient, a colleague, or another program in the system for failure to get better is not an option. These systems are designed to take clinical responsibility for the entirety of a case and to "own" the care of the individual, their family, and the clinical course of treatment. A functioning system holds as truth that the answer to a compelling clinical challenge exists within the system, not outside of it, and certainly not with one individual or program. For this (and other) reasons, systems of care are hard to assemble and almost always in some stage of development. We have learned this in our own careers through three different systems of care. Each had certain strengths and certainly challenges, but without question offered some important lessons to be learned.

We began in the mid-1980s at Charles River Health Management, a for-profit subsidiary of a larger private psychiatric hospital company located in suburban Wellesley, Massachusetts. Nationally, it was a time of enormous growth in psychiatric care, but most importantly, it was the advent of levels of care. We went from a behavioral health system that really had two treatment options (inpatient hospitalization and outpatient individual therapy) to a quasi-system of graduated programming that attempted to meet a patient's need for transition. The goal, most often, was to move an individual out of an acute care setting and back into their home community where treatment was less restrictive and more accessible.

Charles River Health Management started as an offshoot of the larger hospital system with a focus on developing business partnership projects with the Commonwealth of Massachusetts's Department of Mental Health. Program contracts were innovative for the time and carried a promise of a public-private partnership in which the state provided funding and oversight. As a result of a legislative mandate to remove kids from adult inpatient state hospitals, there was a growing focus on developing treatment services for children and adolescents in the care of the Department of Mental Health. These were without question difficult kids, many from challenging homes and all with significant psychiatric symptoms and behaviors.

The center of Charles River Health Management was a repurposed state hospital unit housed on the soon to close grounds of Metropolitan State Hospital. The cavernous hospital was a dilapidated complex that at one time had been a part of the Commonwealth's sprawling mental health system. Our service, named the Metropolitan Adolescent and Family program, housed twenty adolescents, boys and girls, and we worked diligently to stabilize significant psychiatric behaviors. The program was challenged to re-integrate an adolescent as soon as possible into a community-based setting with the goal of providing a more "normal" and hopeful experience. In addition to the hospital, the system included two community-based residential programs located in an urban setting (one designed to provide brief treatment stays, and the other for longer care) and an innovative Family Stabilization Team designed to support families as children reintegrated into their family of origin.

Despite the visionary thinking and the promise of the system, in retrospect, it worked well only a part of the time, but at other times, which felt more common, the system failed to meet the ideals it had been built for. It became apparent that working with children in state care involved a host of political and judicial governmental pressures on almost every case. As clinicians and systems architects, we were limited in our ability to effectively use the system to clinically manage the treatment needs of the adolescents within the system. Other individuals, often from the state and with significant influence, had the final say on the admission of a new patient, when an adolescent we were currently treating could be discharged from one program to another, and general control of where and when any movement or transition could occur. As a result, individual program components of the system found themselves admitting new patients into slots needed for step down to a less restrictive level of care and the system became a holding place for patients in certain levels of care far longer than seems necessary. Adolescents, their families, and program staff grew frustrated. Quickly, the system became gridlocked and, consequently, lost its greatest asset, the promise of flexibility and momentum toward health. Among other things, we learned that a true system of care has to have a free hand to use its resources, the components of the system, to service the patient already in its care.

Choate Health Management was our second venture into a system of care and emerged in the 1990s from a substance use program into a Behavioral Health System of Care. The integration of substance use into mental health services was new thinking at the time and was led in part by Ken Minkoff MD, a thought leader in the treatment of dually diagnosed clients (Minkoff and Cline 2004). Dr. Minkoff believed strongly that integrated treatment was the only effective form of treatment and challenged conventional treatments which often compartmentalized disorders and believed that one "disease" had to be cured before treatment could begin on the second.

It was also an important time of reimbursement change in Massachusetts. Managed Medicaid had roared into the Commonwealth and found many mental health providers unprepared and unwilling to embrace the systemic changes that the new funder demanded. Many behavioral health organizations found themselves at a loss to accommodate the significant changes in length of stay and resistant to the development of levels of care that the new payer required. Across the board, managed Medicaid demanded significantly shorter lengths of stay and the added insult of drastically reduced payments. Predictably, providers scrambled. For many, confronted with the possibility of closing their mental health units, Choate Health Management was seen as a means of saving their program, sometimes a last-ditch effort. Choate Health Management was really two businesses in one. Choate owned some programs outright, including an acute care center, an emergency services team, a respite program, a day program, and an intensive outpatient program. It then grew rapidly as a contract manager capable of managing behavioral health units in general hospitals with the promise of re-energizing struggling services and bringing them into the new era of managed care.

As a system, Choate enjoyed significant growth, particularly on the contract management side of the business. New contracts were added, and the system grew increasingly diverse. In addition to the central emphasis on substance use, an emergency services contract was added, then a number of adult inpatient units, and even, in time, a latency age child unit. While the aggregate seemed to suggest a larger system, the collection of programs was more a loose confederacy only joined contractually. Each program was owned by a separate entity, and for each, the incentives and motives varied. As a result, rather than functioning as an integrated behavioral health system, each participant preferred to focus solely on getting their specific needs met. Programs had little patience with each other and showed limited ability or interest in focusing on functioning as a system. We learned a lot about incentives and the need for a single administrative umbrella in creating a working system of care.

Perhaps the most effective and successful behavioral health system we have ever worked in is Walden Behavioral Care. Centered in Waltham, Massachusetts, Walden opened its doors in 2003 and to this day is not just a complete and functional system of care, but a constantly evolving thought leader in the treatment of eating disorders. Walden began through the closing of a small community hospital and a need to repurpose the remaining hospital plant. The former hospital had a small unit that specialized in eating disorders which became the first Walden program. Walden leadership envisioned a system beyond the former inpatient eating disorders unit and created and meticulously developed an eating disorder specialty system, which has developed and grown for more than fifteen years. Today, it is one of the largest treatment programs for eating disorders in the country. Walden has a fully functioning system of care with distinct programming to meet the needs of patients and families struggling with this serious group of illnesses.

In our opinion, eating disorders provide one of the best examples of a need for a truly integrated mental health solution. Effective management of an eating disorder requires integrating both medical care and specialized behavioral healthcare, particularly in the comorbidities that often accompany an eating disorder. For many patients, medical care is needed to address extreme weight loss and rescue someone from the late stages of starvation. Careful coordination with medical providers is essential to assure viability and once weight loss is stabilized with some progress toward restoration, psychiatric treatment in behavioral health programming must address the underlying thinking and distortion that a person with a significant eating disorder frequently experiences.

Within the first few years of ownership, in addition to its licensed inpatient unit, Walden developed a residential treatment program and a system of community-based programs. All were committed to treat individuals struggling with eating disorders as close to their home community and family as possible, and most importantly, all were committed to working together as a system to ensure movement through a therapeutic treatment episode for a patient and their family in the throes of an advanced eating disorder. Clinicians in the system form treatment teams that operate with a free hand in determining the correct next level of care, and from an organizational standpoint, the system has one administrative umbrella. Walden's leadership communicates a cohesive philosophy of care and has the expectation of all employees that they will come to the table with a willingness to work, not as individual experts, but as a system. At Walden, the system, not an individual talent or a single program, holds a patient and their family.

Today, we are at a crossroads. Large health systems are growing their reach and influence by purchasing smaller providers and following the national disruption of the pandemic, where behavioral health employees work and how they remain connected to each other pose huge challenges. In many respects, it is more essential now that we be cognizant of the organizational lessons of the past as the healthcare landscape and a rapidly changing workforce struggles to find balance. We believe this book is a timely contribution to today's healthcare challenges.

References

Behar, L. (1986). A state model for child mental health services: The North Carolina experience. ChildrenToday, 1593, 16–21.

Broskowski, A. (1991). Current mental health care environments: Why managed care is necessary. *Professional Psychology: Research and Practice*, 22(1), 6–14.

Fisher, D. (1994). A new vision of healing as constructed by people with psychiatric disabilities working as mental health providers. *Psychosocial Rehabilitation Journal*, 17, 67–81.

Fisher, W., Barreira, P., Lincoln, A., Simon, L., White, A., and Sudders, M. (2001). Insurance status and length of stay for involuntary hospitalized patients. *Journal of Behavioral Health Services & Research*, 28(3), 334–346.

Friesen, B. and Koroloff, N. (1990). Family-centered services: Implications for mental health administration and research. *Journal of Mental Health Administration*, 17, 13–25.

Insel, T. (2022). *Healing: Our Path from Mental Illness to Mental Health*. Penguin Publishing Group.

Knitzer, J. (1982). *Unclaimed Children: The Failure of Public Responsibility to Children and Adolescents in Need of Mental Health Services*. Children's Defense Fund.

Minkoff, K. and Cline, C. A. (2004). Changing the world: The design and implementation of comprehensive continuous integrated systems of care for individuals with co-occurring disorders. *The Psychiatric Clinics of North America*, 27(4), 727–743.

Salzer, M. (1997). Consumer empowerment in mental health organizations: Concepts, benefits, and impediments. *Administration in Policy in Mental Health Services Research*, 24, 425–434.

Sluyter, G. (1994). Creating a vision for mental health services. *Administration and Policy in Mental Health Services*, 21, 247–250.

Stroul, B. and Friedman, R. (1986). *A System of Care for Severely Emotionally Disturbed Children and Youth*. Georgetown University Child Development Center National Technical Assistance Center for Children's Mental Health.

1

TOWARD A DEFINITION OF A BEHAVIORAL HEALTH SYSTEM OF CARE

As we look toward the future, due in part to changes in parity law and the swelling of behavioral health service demand following the pandemic, we can anticipate much more growth in health systems. In time, it is expected that many will consolidate into a dominant few, and they, in turn, will exert an enormous influence in healthcare delivery in the United States. Systems of care will define access, quality, and cost in health delivery.

Not surprisingly, in today's world, with the number of health systems we already have, there are many definitions of a system and little agreement as to what constitutes what we refer to as a functioning system of care. Despite that confusion, when you, or a member of your family needs behavioral health treatment, you undoubtedly enter one of these health systems. And with that, you enter with some preconceived and often unspoken expectations of what the system of care will provide for you.

For instance, you might have some sense of how a system in other industries work and because of that have some sort of expectation that the care you receive will be coordinated and that communications will be clear and perhaps most importantly, that one part of the system will work smoothly in coordination with another part of the system. You'll also likely assume that upon entering the system, and for the duration of your treatment experience, that you or your loved one will receive state-of-the-art, high-quality treatment. And if you happen to enter the system for treatment for a specific illness, you might reasonably expect that treatment for that specific illness will occur wholly within the treatment system, ideally with the same committed team or at least with providers who know and trust one another. You expect that a system of care provides some sort of one stop shopping for healthcare.

DOI: 10.4324/9781315177366-2

And, of course, due to the specificity of the illness, should you need to transition through different parts of the system, it would be reasonable to assume that there is consistency and fluidity across the components of the system. You should be able to understand the system and how the components of your care are part of a whole and work together toward the goal of getting you or your family member better. In short, each phase of care should flow logically from one phase of treatment to the next phase until you are recovered. In essence, once you are in the system, you should be in, not reapplying and stepping through yet another front door.

And similarly, you should anticipate, especially with complex disorders, that providers that will treat you within the system have the appropriate training to address your needs, but most importantly, that all have a similar orientation and training to your illness in order to address your needs comprehensively. And just like other industries, you would expect that each service provider you encounter will perform their service to an established standard of care and that there are mechanisms in place to ensure that all treatment will meet or exceed that standard.

And lastly, since we're talking about health and your treatment or the treatment of a loved one, it is more than reasonable to expect that the professionals within the system will talk directly to you and communicate with one another in a clear and direct manner. The same would apply to any time you moved to another setting or level of care: that a provider in one segment of the system will communicate directly to a receiving provider in another program to ensure a smooth transition experience.

But it doesn't work that way. Not even close. Despite most behavioral health systems marketing themselves as a comprehensive healthcare experience, most are woefully inconsistent in meeting many of the basic expectations you might have. And in many cases, these systems completely miss the mark. Despite the staggering growth of healthcare funding and push for the development of systems in the United States, most are operating without a shared definition of a system of care.

In reality, each system is essentially free to make up their own definition of a system and to piece their system together however they see fit. The result is a delivery system today that is often more a fragmented collection of different services provided by a vast array of disconnected providers in treatment settings that often compete with one another. In many respects, given the reality of the behavioral health systems that do exist, it is remarkable that individuals entering these systems do as well as they do. Clearly, we must do better.

For those individuals with more complex illnesses, and certainly for individuals with behavioral health disorders who often struggle with two or even three diagnostic presentations, most treatment experiences fail with the patients and family's expectations of the individual most in need, resulting in experiences that end prematurely, often with great frustration. Their expectation at the beginning of treatment for a high-quality healthcare system is short lived, dissolving into something that feels more like stumbling around in a dark room to find the things you need. Many report that these systems are difficult to understand, lack any operational logic as to how they work to treat their disorder, and are rarely consistent in providing a course of treatment that carries across different providers and locations.

These failures play out in a number of ways. Most often, the providers of care, who have been trained to practice as they believe best, follow their own training and experience, and almost always practice in isolation. The result is a lack of consistency in theoretical approach to such an extent that even with colleagues at hand in the same system treating similar disorders, ideas are not shared. When things become challenging, the provider holding the case is at risk and as the sole responsible person starts to invest their energy into finding ways to off-load or pass the case onto another colleague or organization. When at a loss as to how to overcome the clinical challenge, they are alone as the holder of the problem. A very unpleasant place to be.

Additionally, premature endings are often intermingled with payment issues. Insurance companies with little appetite for behavioral health, pick up on confusion around care planning in systems and make what seem to be reactive determinations about benefits. Particularly with longer-term patients, efforts turn away from investing in an organizational approach to treating the individual to looking for reasons to reduce or deny funding. Further treatment is increasingly challenged with suggestions of treatment resistance, or maybe lack of motivation on behalf of the patient. Sometimes words like "chronic" or "custodial," the boneyard of insurance companies, are introduced into utilization review discussions to limit resources.

We believe that to have a successful treatment experience always requires a multifaceted systemic approach, one that can anticipate the complexities facing a patient and family in need and support the most efficacious treatment course. But it's very complicated to pull off. When it works, these treatment experiences are remarkably positive and can be lifesaving. A functioning system of care has the ability to engage a patient and their family proactively, anticipate obstacles, and best prepare for the success of the next episode of care and recovery.

What is a system of care?

In the 1980s, behavioral health adopted the phrase "system of care" to describe a collection of treatment services working together. Over the next forty years, the definition expanded to the point that today there are many organizations that carry the mantle of "treatment system" or a "system of care" and have some degree of ownership or control over an existing group of programs. The healthcare public likes the idea of a system as it's more encompassing than a stand-alone program, and from a payers viewpoint, a system provides a sense that there is ease of access, consistent treatment across often less expensive levels of care, and pricing. Today, the phrase "system of care" is so popular that most behavioral health organizations freely market themselves as all-encompassing "systems of care" to their prospective patients and payers.

We have found that there are very few behavioral health systems that qualify for the designation of a system as we would define it. We contend that for a number of reasons, most behavioral health systems today simply fail to deliver on their promise of providing a higher order of organization of treatment services and with that lacking, fail even further in their promise of impressive treatment outcomes.

Given the looseness that now accompanies many system definitions, what is a system of care? We propose the following definition:

> A system of care is a constellation of treatment services intentionally designed or developed to work together in a coordinated manner. The function of a system of care is to provide a rational and comprehensive path to recovery for individuals with a particular serious mental or behavioral condition or disorder.

Let's consider the major implications of this definition by reviewing its four components separately:

A constellation of treatment services

It is pretty much a given that any system that treats a serious mental disorder will require a number of services or programs, some delivered at the same time but also some delivered in sequence. Because of the serious nature of the behavioral health disorders that these systems of care are intended to care for, there is usually first a need for an acute care treatment setting. Acute care usually consists of a twenty-four hour (hospital or residential) level of care. In actual practice, most individuals entering the system will, at some point in the course of their treatment, require some intervention from this highest level of care. And, at the other extreme, almost all individuals are going to need some form of ongoing supportive treatment, most often provided in the community and at a minimum, on a weekly basis. But the real innovation that a system of care provides has to do with what happens in the middle, between the acute care setting and outpatient community-based work. This is where levels of transitional services are in place to provide a continuum of services, each designed to effectuate a smooth transition from intensive twenty-four-hour care to intermittent weekly therapy encounters.

Although it is hard to believe today, for many years leading up to the early 1990s, reimbursement for psychiatric and psychological services was only available in two levels of care: inpatient hospitalization and outpatient treatment. In an odd way, that two-tiered "system" created an over reliance on acute care despite it being both the most restrictive and costly level of care. Looking back, it is pretty clear that this occurred because few outpatient clinicians were willing to accept the risk that a discharging inpatient represented, and conversely for many patients, the transition from the security and containment of a twenty-four-hour level of care to such limited outpatient support was too great a treatment step. Often, when such a transition was attempted, failure was commonplace. Many people wound up without any care or shifted from the mental health system to the substance use system, correctional facilities, or even homelessness. While this two-tiered system experienced high levels of growth in the United States, in retrospect, it was adequate for those with moderate behavioral health problems and woefully inadequate for those struggling with serious behavioral health conditions.

The internal logic of a System of Care posits that serious and often debilitating conditions require well-planned services that allow a patient, their family, and even their providers of care to mitigate treatment risk and afford the individuals

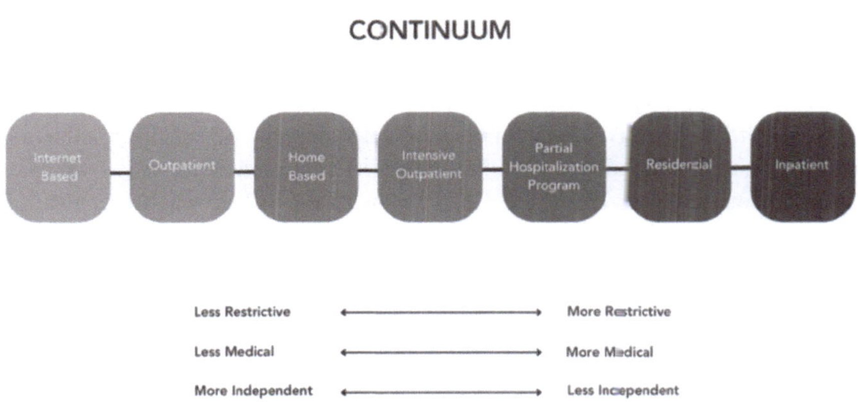

FIGURE 1.1 Linear representation of a System of Care. Sometimes referred to as "Continuum of Care", this illustration depicts a sampling of mental health programs that provide service of varying types and intensities.

Source: Original diagram constructed by the authors.

in treatment a "step-down" to a range of intermediate supports. As a general rule, all transitional levels of care must collaborate to support any move away from acute levels of care by providing "just enough" ongoing support to assist the individual in their recovery process. In the same way that medication may be titrated down as individual conditions improve, systems of care seek to titrate non-pharmacologic therapeutic support through transitional levels of care.

It is also important to add that the programs or components that make up these levels of care in a system are fluid, not rigid. Indeed, creative programming evolves and is an essential aspect of the ever-expanding behavioral health system. We witnessed this firsthand through the recent pandemic. Many behavioral health providers, unable to maintain group and individual programming on site due to restrictions imposed to limit the spread of the virus, creatively changed their models. With limitations on accessing health centers and offices, many moved their onsite programming to virtual platforms. Virtual behavioral health treatment was quite limited for the decade prior to the pandemic for a host of reasons. But the pandemic was a catalyst for change and with limited access and a nationwide scramble for services, state licensing regulations were relaxed, payers got on board and saw the value in easing access and clients, and their families moved seamlessly from office-based interventions to on-screen individual and even group modalities.

Intentionally designed or developed to work together in a coordinated manner

This may seem obvious, but without coordination, a system of care is only marginally better than any group of randomly chosen programs. While this point will be discussed at length in subsequent chapters, the impact of close coordination in a system cannot be overemphasized. It relates directly to the ultimate effectiveness of a system of care. Unfortunately, we see disorganization a lot in behavioral health. It is common for different organizations to own parts of a system, even an entire level of care, with the risk of each organization bringing to the table their own admission criteria, philosophy of care, treatment approach, and most importantly, their own culture. This rarely works smoothly.

We have found that a system's commitment to individual patient coordination is a key ingredient that truly creates the "tailoring" effect of a functioning system. One way to think about this is that the system of care as a whole provides an array of tools, but these tools require a great deal of coordination to make them work uniquely and in a sequence to meet the needs of each individual. It is through this coordination of care that the clinicians within the system are able to step away from their own limited view of a case and determine what program(s) an individual needs at a given time and how to seamlessly access each program.

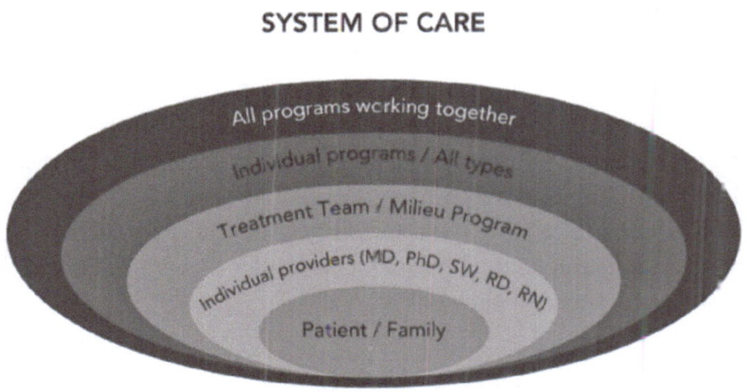

FIGURE 1.2 Patient centric view of a System of Care. In a well-conceived System of Care, the patient and family experience coordinated treatment and support from within and among all of the providers and programs at each level of care.

Source: Original diagram constructed by the authors.

Embedded in this is an understanding of the role that each program in the system plays and when one should begin to consider movement or change in programming to comfortably initiate the next step in a treatment journey.

Providing a rational and comprehensive path to recovery

At its core, the ultimate goal of any system of care is to provide a rational and comprehensive path to recovery. This may seem simplistic, but the truth is that most individuals and their families that struggle with serious behavioral health conditions are often left to fend for themselves and navigate a dense labyrinth of services. Consider their reality; at a time of remarkable vulnerability, a challenged individual is asked repeatedly to navigate a highly fragmented and difficult to understand care system with many programs. Perhaps deliberately, we confuse people even more by describing the system, its components, and treatments by acronyms most people have never heard of. And, if by some stroke of good fortune, an individual finds a program that promises to meet their needs, once in treatment they likely encounter widely disparate clinical philosophies. In their time of greatest need, there is little or no direction.

A thoughtfully conceived system of care is very different. It provides an easy to navigate array of programs that work fluidly and complement each other in such a way as to reinforce the learning and skill acquisition that occurs at each stop along the way. Importantly, how the system works, including entry points, and the anticipated flow through programs in the system are clearly explained in language that an individual and their family can understand. The end of treatment or the goal of moving toward recovery is stated at the entry point along with a definition of recovery that is individually constructed with due consideration given to the patient's own hopes and desires. In general, recovery is, in essence, re-establishing each person's humanity as unique individuals. In the recovery journey, each person is able to voice their values and aspirations that go way beyond the view of them as people with disabilities. In other words, recovery is the process of re-establishing an individual's "personhood" with full acceptance and participation in the world as they envision it.

...for individuals with a particular serious mental or behavioral disorder

The last phrase of our definition is important because it is essential to understand that a system of care works best when it, and everyone who works in it, is focused on the needs of the specific population the system is designed to treat. That's a very important distinction. Today, most behavioral health systems and the behavioral health clinicians employed by them try to treat all comers. There's a certain logic to it; clinicians are often trained as generalists, meaning that their academic and clinical training is thought to apply to a broad spectrum of behavioral health disorders, and most systems look to increase revenue by accepting as many paying customers as possible. This rarely works to the benefit of the consumer.

As behavioral health systems recognize the need to become specialized and focus on a select disorder or cluster of disorders, clinicians entering the system need to explicitly understand which population of users the system of care is designed to care for and implied in that, the specific techniques that are to be used for treatment so that the services are specifically tailored for the needs of that group. This brings the familiar phrase of "patient-centeredness" to a new level. The broader the definition of the population the system says they can serve, the more general the system of care becomes. Providing general or "generic" treatment to a wide variety of patients will reduce the impact of the system. Alternatively, a system that is designed around the needs of a specific population accepts the reality that no system can be all things to all people and allows for and trains its staff to the specificity of treatment modalities needed to address these disorders.

This often gets played out at the point of hire with clinical talent. When the system requires specific treatment modalities, it will increase the need for specialized training. The individual hired into the system must be committed and engaged in meeting the needs of the specific population and in turn be provided with training in the modalities that the system endorses for treatment.

To the extent that a system of care is designed more around the caregivers needs than the users of the services, the effectiveness will be reduced. It is critical to understand that an effective system of care cannot attempt to be "all things to all people."

Lastly, it is important to clarify from the outset that development of a system of care is neither easy nor inexpensive. While it might be possible and good to develop a system of care for a minor condition, the fact is that most of the existing systems of care or pseudo systems of care are attempting to take on major psychiatric disorders and conditions. The costs of these conditions are extremely high in all senses – personal, financial, and to us as a society, and ineffective attempts to provide services to treat these conditions alienate individuals from treatment and are a major driver of the rapid escalation of healthcare costs over the last half century. When considered in this context, the necessary cost of a systems' development makes good clinical and economic sense. Examples of disorders that qualify for this designation include schizophrenia, autism, mood disorders, substance abuse, eating disorders, and a host of others.

Case study: Recovery story – A brief treatment in a system of care

Christina H was fifteen years old when her parents first became concerned about her weight loss. A gifted athlete, she had risen in the ranks of the town's soccer league and had improved so quickly that she was encouraged to play at a higher level, with specialized coaches. While she was honored at the recognition she received, she found the higher level of soccer demanding with its high-intensity practices and demanding level of commitment. Still, she loved the pace of the team. And Christina was an ideal teammate. She was anxious to learn all she could about how to play the game and eager to improve as a player.

One day after practice, she overheard some of the other girls talking about diets. Each seemed enthusiastic about how their diet could improve their athletic performance and each spoke convincingly about how dieting would make them lighter and hence able to run faster. Some even touted results, proudly talking about dropping 2, 3, or even four pounds with seemingly little effort. That night, in the privacy of her room, she did what she always does when confronted with a problem: she went online. Christina found a lot of information about diets.

She was quickly drawn to sites that promised dramatic weight loss in a short period of time. They professed to make weight loss easy, and each offered many tips for success. To her, it was a logical decision; if she really wanted to be a better soccer player, she should lose some weight. Logically, she figured that being lighter on her feet would make her faster on the field. She was sure that success in dieting, just like practicing as a player, would produce quick rewards. With the same commitment and dedication that had helped her excel at soccer, she began that night her new experiment in dieting.

It was difficult at first, but for reasons she didn't understand, with the passing of each day, she felt more driven. Christina initially reduced daily meals from three to two and then figured out ways to secretly not eat all of her remaining two meals. She especially liked that she was in control of what she ate and experienced an almost euphoria when she was most hungry. And the euphoria inspired her to push further. Missing breakfast was easy even with her parents rushing off to work. Mornings always seemed harried anyways with getting to school on time and her parents' preoccupation with their own hectic schedules.

To her surprise, lunch was even easier. She learned how to sit with her friends in the school cafeteria and pretend she was eating, even though she was not. At the end of the lunch period, she would quickly throw away any evidence of her uneaten meal and run off to her next class. Her parents and the teachers at school never knew. Dinner was the biggest challenge. So, she turned again to her friend, the internet, and quickly picked up tricks from other girls her age in the online chat room. Soon, she was an expert on not eating and avoiding the attention of her parents.

With a dramatic decrease in the amount of food she was taking in and the increasing demands of a highly competitive soccer league, her body quickly responded. Christina dropped twenty pounds within five weeks. What she hadn't anticipated was that rather than feel satisfied with her weight loss, she felt disappointed and decided to increase it further still. She pushed herself to eat even less and set new goals. In her mind, she thought incessantly throughout the day about losing weight. She became preoccupied with how thin she could become.

Christina couldn't help but to compare herself to everyone she met. Unexpectedly, the dieting euphoria began to change and rather than feeling exhilarated, things turned dark, and she started to feel a bit frightened, like maybe things were going too fast. It occurred to her one night alone in her bedroom that she was no longer in control, and more frightening than that, she had the sense that she was actually losing control. She went from feeling that she was the master of her diet to maybe it was mastering her.

It was around this time that her parents took notice and became worried. They had been alerted by the mother of one of Christina's friends that other girls were noticing that she was talking too much about food and eating too little. Although their initial thought was that the mother was being intrusive, after a family holiday gathering in which other family members also made comments, what had seemed intrusive parenting became a chorus of concern. Some family members who had not seen Christina in months didn't hold back their worry. In the blunt manner of families, the quiet problem became apparent.

A trip to the pediatrician validated everyone's worst fears. Not only had Christina dropped a significant amount of body weight, but her pulse and blood pressure were dangerously low. Her doctor immediately took a worried tone and he turned very serious. He recommended an inpatient hospitalization for an eating disorder.

Christina hated the hospital. The staff talked too much about the lethality of eating disorders, and with three group meals a day and even snacks between meals, the abundance of food was overwhelming. Every day, Christina was pushed in daily meetings with a Registered Dietician. Her intake slowly increased. Her weight and vital signs were monitored around the clock. And as if to add insult to injury, she was forced to meet with a therapist who wanted to know far more about her life than she had ever told anyone.

Her parents, however, had a different experience. While they felt great relief and learned as much as they could from the staff, they lived in fear of what might come next. They knew firsthand that this is a persistent disorder and while they desperately wanted their daughter back, they remembered well how hard it had been to get her into the hospital to begin with. A family meeting that focused on the idea of a frightening next step heightened their anxiety. The team recommended a step down to the system's residential program. Feeling like war-torn soldiers, the parents pleaded for a longer stay in the hospital. For them, this didn't seem like the time for a change; stability had finally arrived. Besides, they had finally gotten to a place of trusting the treatment team. Any movement seemed like a threat.

Familiar with this response from a family, the treatment team reminded them that they were now in a system of care. They reviewed all the levels of care that are a part of the system and reiterated that a move to another level of care is not a discharge per se, rather a necessary next step in treatment. What seemed to reassure them the most was a commitment that if the move to the residential program did not work, for whatever reason, a quick step up back to the inpatient program would happen. A new admission and admission process would not be required.

The team executed a well-orchestrated hand-off and Christina transferred into the residential program where she remained for a number of weeks. While there, her nutritional progress continued, and through her work in groups and therapy, she gained some tools to better manage her eating disordered thoughts and insight into the role they had played in her life. She felt stronger and was discharged to an Intensive Outpatient Program near her home. She attended the program three evenings a week with at least one of her parents.

They were one of many families in the program and each program evening Christina was weighed and a discussion ensued about what she had eaten and how she was feeling. The gains she made in the residential program stabilized and slowly, now as an outpatient, she added more weight. After a number of weeks, she was discharged from the Intensive Outpatient Program to an outpatient therapist who worked closely with her pediatrician. A few months later, her soccer career resumed, although this time at a more tempered pace. Christina is an eating disorder success story.

2

PROPERTIES OF A BEHAVIORAL HEALTH SYSTEM OF CARE

In the ever-evolving landscape of healthcare delivery, the need for efficient organizational structures cannot be overstated. Organizational structures play a pivotal role in shaping the functioning and effectiveness of a system. Understanding the them within a system is paramount for optimizing resource allocation, enhancing patient outcomes, and ensuring operational efficiency. One commonly observed organizational structure within healthcare systems of care is the hierarchical model. This structure typically features a clear chain of command, with decision-making authority flowing from the top down. This is very evident in a hospital setting with a CEO at the helm, followed by department heads, managers, and frontline staff. This hierarchical arrangement fosters clarity in roles and responsibilities, streamlines communication channels, and facilitates efficient resource allocation. However, critics argue that rigid hierarchies can impede innovation, hinder interdisciplinary collaboration, and create barriers to effective communication (Essex et al. 2023). Some healthcare systems adopt a matrix organizational structure in which individuals report to both functional managers (e.g. department heads) and project managers simultaneously (Allcom 1990). This is thought to allow for cross-functional collaboration and specialization. Matrix structures are particularly prevalent in interdisciplinary settings such as outpatient clinics or research institutions, where teams often work across traditional departmental boundaries. While matrix structures promote flexibility and expertise utilization, they can also lead to role ambiguity and power struggles if not managed effectively (Burns 1989).

DOI: 10.4324/9781315177366-3

An increasingly popular approach within healthcare systems of care is the network organizational structure. This model emphasizes collaboration and interdependence among various entities, including hospitals, primary care practices, community organizations, and social services agencies. The hope is that networks facilitate seamless care coordination, information sharing, and resource pooling, ultimately enhancing patient-centric care delivery (Provan et al. 2003). However, managing diverse stakeholders within a network can pose challenges related to governance, accountability, and standardization of care protocols (Evans et al. 2024).

There's a story in the Old Testament about the building of a tower as a way of honoring God. The tower was to be so tall that it would achieve what no other structure had achieved: to reach beyond the clouds to the heavens. Word went out to neighboring countries about this great and noble effort. Soon people from faraway lands, hearing of the great challenge, began to arrive, almost as if they were drawn to the site to help. Despite the best of intentions, what ensued was somewhat of a construction nightmare.

The convergence of people, with no shared language or vision, found it nearly impossible to plan and communicate with one another. One construction crew could not talk to another and even ideas of how to actually build the tower could not be expressed nor put into action. In fact, there were lots of arguments about who should even be in charge. Despite the best of intentions, no meaningful information was shared, and disagreements grew. Each team was left trying to build the tower by themselves in the way that they saw fit. Ultimately, there was a crash of biblical proportions and the entire effort failed.

The story is named the Tower of Babel (Genesis 11: 1–9), and it's a story which highlights among other things the critical role of organization, planning, and communication. As with all biblical stories, there is a lesson to be learned and one of the lessons learned from the Tower of Babel is that a shared vision is an essential vehicle for true cooperation, and mechanisms must be in place to facilitate collaboration among people in any significant undertaking. In many ways, our current behavioral health system is a modern-day Tower of Babel. Patients and families, often in the midst of crisis, are faced with a significant behavioral health need and are drawn to an institution or a system that offers them a sense of hope for a cure or at least, a start on the road to recovery. They come seeking an understanding of what the presenting problem is, and most importantly, a direction forward that promises to be an attempt to heal. What patients and their families often find is a communication cacophony of biblical proportions. They find that healthcare is a modern nightmare with no shared vision and where one provider often does not understand another provider even in the same organization.

We believe that in order for a system of care to function and be effective, it must be constructed according to certain rules or pillars, similar to the posts and beams that support the structure of a building. In our structure of a behavioral health system, each pillar plays an important role. It provides a critical element of support like the supports that hold up a well-constructed building. In both cases, all the supports are essential because the weight of the structure must be equally distributed across all the pillars, creating a sense that the building, or in this case, system, is structurally sound. In essence, each pillar provides a core element essential to the working system of care and each contributes a critical component that is needed to reduce a natural tendency for fragmentation.

The pillars we will present are applicable to any behavioral health system regardless of service specialization. This means that they apply to both the systems that treat individuals with a variety of mental illnesses as well as emerging specialty systems which might focus more specifically on mood disorders, substance use, or eating disorders. While all healthcare organizations aspire to have a sound structure that creates a healing environment, the development of a sound structure takes time and is a significant investment of resources. And realistically, it is always a work in progress. As we introduce each pillar, it is important to notice the complexity of each (some of which will be further developed in later chapters of this book) and the significant effort needed to coordinate the whole. In many respects, building a system according to these pillars and then monitoring each and making adjustments over time is the most important work of the organization. It is work that is never completed.

The pillars of our system are:

Pillar 1 A single administrative umbrella
Pillar 2 Leadership
Pillar 3 A shared clinical philosophy and approach
Pillar 4 Shared responsibility and accountability
Pillar 5 Consistent operational practices

Although it is to be expected that some of the pillars we present may vary in their degree of sophistication at any time given the development of an organization, it is important to note that all are essential and require a significant degree of planning by the organization's leadership to implement and to ensure that all are in practice simultaneously. Once implemented, it is the job of leadership to provide ongoing (and even relentless) oversight to ensure that the principles of each become ingrained into the fabric of the organization's culture and ultimately translate into the treatment experience of each patient and family.

We have found that absent daily attention to the details of each pillar by the organization's senior leadership, the collective support that these pillars represent to the system will quickly deteriorate. It is important to say that this can occur almost organically and seemingly without notice. We have found that shifting of each pillar can occur not out of malice or neglect but rather due to the numerous challenges facing each program in the organization and the often-prevailing demands of day-to-day operational exceptions, often made by well-meaning managers and clinicians. For example, a staffing crisis or a challenging new admission may initiate a change or workaround in hiring or training. This is especially true at the critical points of care progression, moving from one program to another, for a patient and family as they work their way through the system. Rigorous oversight by senior leadership ensures that the system works as it was designed, and, to be successful, leadership is required to have a sustained focus, ongoing and repetitive training, and above all, patience.

Pillar 1: A single administrative umbrella

In truth, many behavioral health systems today are systems in name only. At best, they are a loose confederation of programs that come together from competing organizations to strategically join services to address a business need. They create a collection of services or programs that tend to be aligned around some core administrative functions, for instance: admissions, human resources, billing, IT, and training, and each has the goal of creating efficiencies. From the outside, especially to potential patients, their families, and insurance payers, each of these systems looks like a functioning system. What people see is an array of behavioral health programs cleverly marketed together to create the perception of one stop shopping and continuity in behavioral health services. A client or family in need of care enters with great hopes and a degree of confidence.

Of course, both are short lived, and once the veil is lifted, the problems are glaring. These systems are unclear in the lines of leadership and as a result fail to operate with the necessary authority to regulate the system. They are not just fragmented, they never worked as a whole. No one individual or group of leaders holds real authority, and as a result, the system fails to perform according to the clinical vision needed to provide a healing treatment experience. And to make matters worse, any authority that does exist is often delegated to lower-level managers who are ill equipped to negotiate the intentions of each participating partner. As a result, the advantages that the "system" is supposed to bring get lost in a hodgepodge of cultures and lack of clinical direction. These systems fall woefully short of the client's expectations many times, resulting in a disrupted treatment experience or worse, a frustrating and precipitous ending to treatment.

A single administrative umbrella changes all that and is the distinguishing difference between these quasi-systems and what we would identify as a truly functioning system. A single administrative umbrella is a dramatic visual which depicts the reach and power of an organization's authority and capacity over the entirety of the system. We believe an administrative umbrella is a critical element needed to carry out the clinical vision of the system and specifically to control the levers of management needed to make the system "behave like a system" rather than a group of independent interests. In essence, an administrative umbrella is the single greatest force against fragmentation for a system, and without it, most programs will inevitably veer off course.

Lacking a single administrative umbrella, programs lose any chance of a cohesive vision and develop an unspoken "groupthink" between the local managers and their staff. Central authority is avoided and gets played out in a variety of ways, most common being arguments between programs in the system about the type of patient that seems to be the best "fit" for each program as well as the type or profile of patients that should be excluded entirely from entering treatment. Even with the best of intentions, a program's "groupthink" can justify to internal employees and even other programs why it should operate outside of the parameters of the larger system. It is easy to lose sight of how or why, as a specific service, it should contribute to the larger system of care.

With no direct communication and connection to the larger system, a local program leader will begin to think of their program similarly to that of a small franchise. The larger system becomes secondary as the local manager is faced with many daily challenges, including fluctuations in census, staffing shortages, and clinical fidelity. Local managers struggle for survival and tend to solve problems themselves. They anticipate that they cannot look to other programs in the system for help when it is needed and as a result look for the solution to their daily challenge, whether that be a staffing shortage or in managing a difficult patient, from within their program. They become psychologically separated from the whole and resource poor in the system, thinking of themselves as independent fighters struggling to address their own needs rather than members of a collective with resources to share based on need. Programs will inevitably begin to vary from one another and will become more and more independent of the larger organization. Silos, a hallmark of healthcare, develop quickly. From the patient's perspective, the possibility of a productive treatment episode erodes and can be heard through complaints about different admission criteria, inconsistencies in treatments even within a single program, and mismanaged and abrupt transitions from one level of care to another.

Case study

A large community health center had just been awarded a state contract that created a new revenue stream to service high-need individuals in the care of the state. It seemed like an easy implementation for the health center. They created partnerships with several other local organizations to meet the obligations of the contract, each controlling one of the programs described. Under one roof, though administered by three different organizations, was an emergency services team, an outpatient clinic, and a well-regarded day treatment program. Remarkably, months after implementation, individuals in charge of the care for the cohort of state consumers complained that they couldn't access the services they felt they needed for their members. Some of those services were even in the same building.

Why such an access problem existed and more importantly, how to correct it became the topic of discussion at a senior management meeting. Interestingly, the problem between programs had risen to the senior administrator's attention not as a clinical concern (they were unaware that there even was a problem) rather as a revenue problem with projections for increased revenue in the newly contracted program not being realized. Despite the promise of easy access to services co-located in the same building, it became clear that something was wrong with the partnership. There was no free movement of patients from one organization to another: no flow. The group learned that each program in the building had set their own admission criteria and in the process of an admission included a screening procedure that excluded many in the new cohort at the front door of treatment.

There was indignation that the staff was not working together and of course a fair amount of finger pointing. "What is wrong with those people?" one senior administrator queried. Blame was liberally directed to the program supervisors in each program as well as leadership in the partnering organizations. What was absent was any awareness from the senior administrators that they may have played a role in the problem. As a group, and ultimately as an organization, they failed to create a single administrative umbrella. Unable to speak with a clear authoritative voice across the group of programs, it was impossible to maintain a focus on the basic operational procedures. At the end of the day, despite working in proximity, the programs failed to meet the needs of the clients they served.

We find this often in larger organizations which develop portfolios of related businesses often because of environmental opportunities rather than strategic planning. Organizational changes such as a merger, an acquisition, or even bankruptcy can escalate the process. It is essential in the early stages of such developments to create an administrative umbrella, one voice that can move the organization when needed and ensuring that programs are operating to the goals of the system rather than the needs of local ownership, managers, and staff.

Case study

A small human service agency quickly doubled in size due to an opportunistic merger with a much larger but struggling organization. The host leadership team quickly went from a small functioning group with good operational oversight and a high degree of program-specific knowledge to a stretched team with little knowledge of their newly acquired business. They had become seduced by their newfound size and enjoyed the influence they now had in the area's behavioral health landscape. With eyes wide, they envisioned an even larger, more powerful organization, and their dreams of influence grew even more.

They moved their focus away from program operations to program growth and, of course, it came at a cost. The team quickly found that their management experience with their smaller organization was of limited utility when matched to a now larger organization. They realized that they had much less control of their newly acquired portfolio of programs and with all the attention that it demanded, their core business began to suffer. Of necessity and not knowing what else to do, they made a decision to move away from their tight oversight of programs and delegated as much responsibility as possible to local program managers.

While some program managers welcomed this change, many experienced the shift in senior leadership's attention with some apprehension. Managers in each program now felt a need to protect themselves and their program during this time of transition and as a result started to think locally rather than as a part of a larger working system. Losing sight of their interrelatedness, the programs quickly fragmented. Even the goal of being a system of care, something they were all proud of, changed. Without the administrative mechanisms and the vigilant attention of leadership in place to assure consistent program performance, their interrelatedness waned as each program developed a sense of fierce independence.

Over time, local programs created their own preferred client base and with it a growing list of clients they would, or would not, treat. Treatment protocols that had been widely accepted across the system were altered based on the skills and preferences of the program staff and even the interests and talents of newly hired team members. The smooth transitions from one level of care to another became a thing of the past as it became harder and harder to make a referral to another program. Applications for admission began to emerge in which clients were screened for appropriateness and compatibility with the talents of the staff. Organizational culture, once a collaborative experience, grew so hostile that even co-located programs despite proximity and a shared client base refused to work together to manage admissions and sick calls.

In a behavioral health system structured with a single administrative umbrella, this cannot happen. A single administrative umbrella assures that all the employees who work in the system are responsive to one administrative structure and therefore buy into a shared vision for behavioral health treatment. It creates a boundary around a system of care and a set of specific system rules that clearly define whom the system is prepared to treat (as well as who the system is not designed for), the specific program components of the system, how treatment in each program, or level of care, will be delivered, and how the levels of care and specific programs relate to each other.

Pillar 2: Leadership

Our second pillar emphasizes the role that leadership plays in creating a functioning behavioral health system. Leadership is critical in any organization but especially in behavioral health due to the intensely personal nature of the work. This gets played out in both informal and formal leadership. Informal leadership exists to some degree in each employee in the organization and for that reason is far reaching in its ability to influence an organization to the good and to its detriment. Informal leadership is the ability of an individual or group of people to influence, usually through their own interpersonal skills, the thinking, motivation, and activity of those around them. In a system of care, this can be quite powerful when used in a positive manner. It's the employee who really commits to the mission of the system and who, through their work example, can influence those around them in a positive way. These are the people who are invaluable in creating a dynamic team spirit and certainly the people to develop and retain.

Of course, informal leadership can go in the opposite direction, to the detriment of an organization. These can be an employee or a group of employees who not only do not buy into the vision and mission of an organization but often use their skills to spread negativity and discontent. Though maybe not always aware, they tend to use their influence to undermine the organization. These are people who never seem satisfied with an organization's efforts and are suspicious of initiatives from system leadership. Negative informal leaders can be dangerous if they are successful in spreading their discontent and they do so by finding or building a larger group in which to sway. When negative informal leaders gain followers, they can become very powerful and have the potential of creating a cancer that can spread throughout an organization. They can undo the work of many good employees.

Formal power, however, is quite different. These are designated leaders in an organization, and each has the ability to exert the authority of their position across the organization. They can move or direct the organization in a certain direction. In most behavioral health organizations, formal leadership often occurs through the person of the Chief Executive Officer and selected senior administrators. While there is much written about the qualities needed to make these formal leaders effective in their roles, there is no template or litmus test for a truly great CEO. There are however some distinctive qualities that make a CEO an effective leader in a system of care and in our experience, we identify the following as critical qualities.

First, the CEO must be an individual who holds a strong professional and personal belief that systems of care are the best means for delivering healthcare. They must be true system thinkers. While many people can expound on how much they know about systems and even tout experience working in other systems, an exceptional CEO believes to their core that a well-functioning system of care is, without question, the best and only way to provide effective treatment and to achieve recovery in behavioral health. In fact, these leaders must feel so strongly about a system of care as the model for behavioral health delivery that should the need arise, they would elect to have a member of their own family or close friend in need of treatment treated in a system of care. In fact, they would likely choose their system. They have an unwavering belief that treatment in the system is superior to treatment in any other setting, even from a well-regarded stand-alone program or from a highly talented and respected individual practitioner.

Second, a great CEO must be something of a benevolent dictator. We have encountered many who are either affable politicians or to the other extreme, insensitive taskmasters. Neither really works. But a benevolent dictator is an individual who can engage personally with people in the organization and communicates an enthusiasm for the creative healing efforts that the system provides. This is the benevolent part. This same individual must also be able to unapologetically demand that the programs in the system and the staff members in each program work together at all times to the benefit of their patients and the system. As the ultimate success of the system is contingent on getting program staff from one program to work in unison with the program staff from another program, the benevolent dictator CEO must charismatically engage and market employees in that effort ("you really want to do this"), while at the same time insisting that the system operate true to its vision ("in this organization, this is how we work. If you are to work here, you must do it this way"). The exceptional CEO can visualize how the system optimally should work and is more than willing to use their formal authority to make the people in the system respond to that vision in a clear, unified direction.

Third, the CEO is charged with positioning the system to meet the anticipated and unanticipated changes that rapidly occur in the healthcare marketplace. These are the unpredictable waters of healthcare and we experienced this firsthand during the recent pandemic.

Case example

With the abrupt arrival of Covid-19, things happened quickly and like most services in healthcare, we found ourselves facing a changed world almost overnight. With no advance warning and little time for preparation, basic health information impacting our patients and staff seemed to shift daily. A protocol implemented one day was altered sometimes the very next day with little guidance from either our state or federal regulators. Fear and anxiety grew. We quickly realized that we couldn't get our patients to our outpatient programs or staff members coming to work in our twenty-four-hour programs unless we could provide some degree of safety assurance. Many were fearful that by coming to work and having contact with others that they would spread the virus to their homes and loved ones. It was a time of great fear and uncertainty, and there was a distinct need for the CEO and senior leadership to step in.

What happened was nothing short of remarkable. In short order, leadership banded together and took charge. Our outpatient leaders were charged with developing virtual programming, a task they enthusiastically undertook, and the equipment needed was quickly deployed to staff members in their homes. In one weekend (albeit a long one), program leaders were able to put together the structure for virtual outpatient programming that developed in sophistication over the weeks that followed. The opportunity to work from home was enthusiastically received by fellow employees and our patients. And in our twenty-four-hour programs, protective supplies and testing were quickly procured along with creative temporary housing arrangements for those who felt the need to remain separate from family for a period of time.

For all our employees, a weekly town meeting was convened to impart information and to hear concerns. These meetings allowed our employees to see a leadership that was visible and engaged. The ability of our leadership to communicate directly and with transparency to all employees instilled a sense of confidence and a belief in the organization. Information was transparent with infection numbers openly shared along with clear steps that were taken to implement protective protocols from the Centers for Disease Control. There was honest talk about people's fears and concerns and while we struggled with conflicting information at times, there was comfort in knowing that our leadership could be trusted and were watching out for our collective best interests. Through the experience, we came together as an organization.

And last, we have found that having practicing behavioral health clinicians serving in senior leadership roles is a great advantage. While some might think that this is not a wise business decision and express concern that clinicians will perform poorly when faced with the business aspects of healthcare, we've found just the opposite. Experience has taught us that it is probably easier to train a talented clinician to be a good manager (and to understand business principles) than it is to hire a businessperson and ask them to understand the work of behavioral health through the eyes of a clinician.

We often speak a mantra that good clinical care is good business and vice versa, that we hold the clinical mission and the business mission of the organization to be co-equal, and with some training and support, have found our clinician/leaders capable of balancing their ability to make sound clinical decisions with good business decisions. In our most recent organization, behavioral health clinicians represented over half of the Executive Committee and most of the Senior Leadership team. By using trained clinicians in our leadership structure, we communicate to our workforce that the work we do with people is important and that clinical thinking and values go into every decision, even business decisions. And, importantly, our clinician leaders are all involved in treating patients. We believe that ongoing clinical practice allows our leadership to stay in touch with the real work of the organization. As one senior leader said, "we want to go home at the end of the day being aware of that anxiety that accompanies working with a challenging client or a difficult clinical decision. It keeps us focused on the importance of our work."

Case example: Program directors and business decisions

Program staff in our acute care facility were engaged in treating a sixteen-year-old adolescent who had been admitted for suicidal ideation. In learning about the case, it became clear that the adolescent was struggling with a longstanding and recently escalated conflict with her mother. One of our clinicians met several times with the mother and daughter during the hospitalization to address their conflict and some progress was made. Fortunately, the state's child protection agency had recently become involved and was willing to place the adolescent outside of the home for an additional period in the hopes that some more family work might mitigate the conflict and allow for a safe return home.

While treatment was progressing, the insurance payer became concerned with the length of stay and in what seemed to be an impulsive decision, the payer denied further payment for the acute care stay. This decision put the treatment team in a bind. They knew the adolescent and mother would need time to prepare for a change in level of care and the child protective agency would not be able to respond immediately with adequate placement. The treatment team struggled with discharging the adolescent back to her mother in a move that felt precipitous, or holding the adolescent for some additional days until the state agency could secure a less restrictive out-of-home placement. It was clear that holding the adolescent at the acute care setting would be a financial loss for the hospital as the extended stay would not be covered by the insurer.

After some discussion with the treatment team and the Chief Operating Officer, the Program Director made the decision to keep the adolescent in the acute care setting and not to discharge. The financial risk to the program was mitigated by initiating an appeal with the insurance company for any lost revenue, and at the same time, the program worked to prioritize the case for the state agency. The Program Director's decision felt like the right thing to do for the program staff and was supported within the organization.

The critical role of local leadership

We rely heavily on local leaders to manage sites across our system. These individuals are usually developed through the system and almost all have worked directly as clinicians under the direction of a senior leader. Most have participated in an in-house management training program and importantly buy into the philosophy of the organization and have an enthusiasm for the work we do. All our local leaders understand that their work is a "ministry of presence," meaning that their onsite visibility and example is paramount to local employees and is ultimately tied to the success of the site.

As the organization grows so does the number of sites in the system and with that growth comes the challenge of distance from the home office or center. Sometimes, this might be a few miles across town, or even the state, but for larger regional systems, the distance can be hundreds and even thousands of miles. With increasing distance comes the risk that local managers will become disconnected from the core leadership or home base of the system. Maintaining open communication and personal contact to assure consistency in programming becomes a significant challenge for the local program manager and senior leadership. This translates into the importance of building supportive relationships among leaders of all levels.

We make a concerted effort to connect local leadership and to keep local leaders connected to the organization's home. This occurs somewhat routinely through structured meetings and communications but most effectively through interventions that are designed to foster connections with other local leaders and senior leadership. For instance, we insist that rather than using email as a primary source of communication, program directors call each other and speak directly to one another. Certainly, email is a tool for scheduling a meeting or passing on bits of information but rarely helps build a relationship. One effective strategy we use is an informal rule that anytime an email exchange exceeds two exchanges, it is time to end emailing one another and to have an in-person call. Though useful, email is a blunt instrument that easily miscommunicates an unintentional tone from one person to another. Speaking directly to a person is essential in building a connection particularly in the event of a disagreement or a feeling of tension.

We also create formal events, like a monthly meeting in which we make every effort to get all local leaders in a room or a Zoom room. It is an opportunity for people to hear and question new initiatives or changes in the system, but the real magic happens before the meeting starts or during a break. We want our leaders not to just know one another but to like one another. And lastly, we use off-site and after-hours events periodically to get people away from work and in a more relaxed atmosphere, like a dinner at a nice restaurant. Although some may criticize this as an unnecessary expenditure, we have found that it pays off in the relationships that are built. Without question, getting people out of the office and into a relaxing atmosphere creates an opportunity for our leaders to get to know each other as people. It is these times that connections are built that make the day-to-day management of programs around the system easier.

Pillar 3: A shared clinical philosophy and approach

Entering a system of care in the context of a significant behavioral health crisis is a devastating experience for a patient and their family. Systems are complicated and confusing even before you add the emotion of an illness. Almost all systems will confuse a family who inevitably become frustrated with what appears to be disjointed programming, forms, delays, and their own exhaustion. Imagine being bombarded with a cacophony of information about services you've never heard of before, many of which are referred to by acronyms that you don't understand.

Most of us are much more familiar with medical systems. We were likely born in one and almost by default have had episodic experience with one or more over years. In some sense, we know when we might need to go to one, and once there, we know basically what to expect. And, in the event that something was to go wrong, we might even know who to appeal to or where an alternative source of help might be. But not so in behavioral health. Most Americans have never touched a behavioral health system and even those who might have needed one likely have gone to great lengths to avoid the experience. When a patient and family present for the first time, it is likely because all other options have been exhausted and the patient and family feel as though they have absolutely no choice. And so, they arrive with terribly stigmatized notions of behavioral health, fearful of the very institutions in which they are seeking treatment.

A functioning Behavioral Health System of Care will almost always present better and ultimately perform better for a family if it is clearly explained to a family at the point of first contact. It is important that the system of care has a logical clinical philosophy that can be simply explained and clearly demonstrated in practice. In short, the system must make sense even during such an emotional time as an admission. In our experience, families may be initially confused about using levels of care as they have not experienced a system that holds a patient through an entire treatment episode. Once explained, however, a system can seem logical and there is a sense of relief in knowing that there is a comprehensive plan in place.

To make sense, the patient and family must grasp that movement or progress in treatment occurs through each level of care and that linear, successive progress is often not expected. They must hear early on that for more serious illnesses we will anticipate movement both forward to less restrictive levels of care and when needed back to more acute levels. They have to hear clearly that the expectation that moving back to a more acute level of care in the continuum is not a failure, rather a needed step to support the patient through a phase in treatment. Moving in and out of levels of care is treatment.

As a part of sharing our approach with patients and families, we are sensitive to the overuse of jargon and acronyms in behavioral health. In many respects, we have developed our own language that while familiar to those of us who work in the field, is unknown to families and patients as they enter the system. What may seem intuitive and efficient communication to our staff comes off as insensitive and needlessly confusing. Simply stated, if the language used to describe the system of care carries no immediate meaning to a patient and their family in the context of a stressful admission, it invariably creates distance at the worst moment.

Additionally, a great system of care has a clinical philosophy that is informed by current research which is known and practiced within the system. This clinical philosophy must be clear and understandable and hold an intuitive logic that inspires confidence that this system may really be able to help. As important, the clinical philosophy must make sense internally to the behavioral health providers who choose to work in the system. Although the techniques or approaches endorsed by the system do not need to be exclusive (they are often a collection of different approaches), it is imperative that each is research informed and can be applied to the illnesses that are to be treated within the system. And importantly, once in place, they must be established and consistently practiced throughout the entire system. It is an organizational expectation that everyone must follow. Unless all providers in the system are trained and monitored in the identified clinical philosophy, treatment practices will erode as clinicians veer away from the organization's clinical approach into their own preferred treatment practices. This happens often unintentionally, with an ebb and flow as clinicians leave the system and new ones join.

Pillar 4: Shared responsibility and accountability

Perhaps one of the greatest learnings for clinical staff in a behavioral health system is the notion that the system, not an individual clinician or single program, is responsible for an outcome. If this is really assimilated into practice, the change can be enormous, but it is complicated. While it might seem a welcome relief to a clinician, for most, the idea of a shared responsibility for a challenging case is counter to their training. Most clinicians are trained as generalists and as such are indoctrinated with the belief that they should be capable of treating almost any patient. And with that, as the holder of the patient, is the burden that they alone are responsible for the outcome. If things go well, a clinician feels empowered and likely attributes success to their talent, but when it doesn't, or in the case of a clinically complex presentation, the clinician is overmatched, and things fall apart.

Every behavioral health system has individuals who present with high-intensity challenges and some aspect of elevated risk. These individuals are often well known in treatment circles as they tend to bounce from one system to another or once in a system, from one provider to another provider. It seems that finding the right system or clinician for treatment becomes an impossible challenge. This plays out each time they enter a system, often to the chagrin of the Admissions Department. Most likely, they find their way to the most acute level of care, and at some point, early in the treatment episode, it becomes clear to all those involved that this individual is far more complex than anticipated. Almost immediately, the focus turns from treatment to moving them out of the system. Discharge becomes the goal with no viable outpatient options and the possibility that actual treatment could occur diminishes. There is rarely talk of recovery and with risk increasing over time, no one wants to be the last one assigned to a patient with a looming bad outcome. Given the lack of care integration most systems struggle with, these individuals are more "managed" than treated and once discharged from the system end up on some sort of "do not admit list." Having shared responsibility alleviates any individual's concern to some degree and allows for the system to persevere with complex patients.

Our fourth pillar addresses this critical component of clinical responsibility; individual practitioners or even distinct programs cannot be solely responsible for a patient. For treatment to occur for a challenging clinical presentation, it is essential that an entire system participates, and that the responsibility be shared across the system. Conceptually, the burden of risk shifts from the individual practitioner or local program to the larger system of care.

This is uncharted practice in behavioral health. Practitioners must be trained out of their independent practice mindset and check their own need to succeed on their own with every patient. Interestingly, when clinical responsibility for a patient's outcome shifts from the individual practitioner or program to a system, things do change. With clinical responsibility shared by all clinicians and programs in the system of care, a path forward emerges. Stated another way, when any patient is admitted into a system of care, no single person or program should be seen as the sole author of the cure. The magic for recovery lies within the workings of the system and a patient's success (or failure) is not tagged to any one individual.

Case example: Selective admissions

A large behavioral health system directed potential patients toward their programs located in a number of outpatient clinics across the state. Each clinic had its own admission procedure and different staff members at each site were delegated to conduct assessments and manage admissions for each day of the week. These assigned admission clinicians pre-screened presenting individuals for their appropriateness for the outpatient program and if the patient was deemed a good fit, they were scheduled for a first appointment in the next available slot.

Where it became a bit cloudy was when the patient was not deemed appropriate for the clinic. In those situations, the patient was sent home with instructions to wait for a call back, often without explanation. When a call to the patient's home eventually came, often two or three days later, the potential patient was instructed to present for yet another evaluation, but this time at a different program. The subtle (or not too subtle) message to the patient was that they had failed in their evaluation and were hence unwanted at the program.

If the patient showed up for their next appointment (which was unlikely), they would undergo another admission process which was very similar to the first. From the patient's perspective, the message was clear; they are not held nor wanted by the program or system in any way. In fact, to the patient seeking support, the process felt directionless. The probability of getting admitted into the system would likely vary depending on the location of the program and even the day of the week and assigned staff member with whom they happened to interact.

Case example

One of our programs was struggling with the transition of a very challenging patient from one level of care to another. The patient's name was Emily, and she was well known throughout the local area due to the high degree of suicidal behavior she frequently presented with in one of the regions' emergency departments. As with any challenging patient, most systems, and even within our own system, some programs, would prefer not to admit Emily. Program Directors became adept at finding reasons to justify why Emily's presentation did not fit with their local level of care. And with almost every attempt to engage in a step-down program, Emily was blocked. She was a "hot potato" who by history has moved from program to program, often in rapid succession. Programs were afraid of her.

For Emily, this came to a crisis point at the time of discharge from our acute level of care. The intended next step was to one of the system's partial hospitalization programs. Despite a successful inpatient admission, her challenging history followed her. Her history of very serious suicidal acts was well remembered, and this time, the insurance company added their voice to the mix of anxiety. They expressed frustration at paying for repeated acute admissions with seemingly limited success. A conference call was convened with leadership from the acute care service, the planned partial hospitalization program that was reluctant to accept her, and the insurance company. In what turned out to be a spirited call, the insurer made the case that they had determined that Emily was not at a point where she could truly utilize any further services. They seemed to have decided that she was unmotivated at the present time and due to that, further treatment was denied.

That surprising pronouncement, coupled with the partial hospitalizations anxiety at accepting her into their program, led the partial hospital program director to propose that Emily should leave the acute care program and discharge home until she was "ready" for treatment. Fortunately, a senior leader saw this as an attempt to exit a challenging patient from the system and intervened. The leader insisted that Emily remain within the system and challenged all involved to rethink the discharge plan to include treatment in the partial hospitalization program (albeit with some additional support).

The review of Emily's care and the careful review of the decision-making behind it led to a larger internal discussion on the system's commitment to caring for challenging individuals over extended periods of time. Most importantly, it afforded the opportunity to reiterate a core principle of the system that often impacts the admission process: that not any individual or program holds complex and challenging patients in isolation. Rather, it is the system that makes a commitment to these individuals, holds them through their course of care, and can allocate additional resources to support a program when necessary. With a more viable plan in place, the insurance company rethought their stance. They agreed to fund the next level of care and the additional support needed to ensure the success of the step down.

Pillar 5: Consistent operational practices

Even with the best clinical philosophy and leadership, as systems grow, there is an almost exponential increase in operational complexity. The task of monitoring to ensure that all sites are practicing in a consistent manner and most importantly, that the system is doing what it is designed to do looms large. Inevitably, variability emerges between programs and the on the ground challenge becomes maintaining a balance between the core practice points that define the system of care and a legitimate need to accommodate the nuances of local geography and culture. Our fifth pillar speaks directly to this task. With a fully functioning system of care, there is a need to identify and define certain essential operational practices that will define the system and then to monitor carefully each of those practices across the system. And there must be a recognized leader who can step in when needed to hear a debate between treatment teams or programs and decide on a next step.

The choice of key transition points can vary with each system of care but all should be selected thoughtfully as they will reflect the values of the system and will be the mechanism to monitor how the system performs. In our own system, we identified three: the point of admission, the experience of a transition between one level of care to another (we refer to this as the hand-off), and last, the point of discharge. Each bears discussion:

A Admission: Most patients and families entering a healthcare system will tell you that they can vividly recall the day they were admitted. If things went well, it is more than likely that the goodwill earned will positively influence the rest of the treatment experience, and if things didn't go well, not only is it a bad indicator of treatment success, but it becomes enormously difficult to turn the experience around so that things start to feel positive. For people in a behavioral health crisis, the point of admission is a critical juncture. We describe it to our staff as one of the more stressful days in the life of a patient and their family. They are inevitably exhausted, frustrated, and while potentially a bit hopeful, likely anticipate being disappointed. Anything that can be done to decrease the degree of stress they feel and to increase confidence in the system is critical for success.

B The Hand-off: It's an odd thing about healthcare in general, but seems especially true in behavioral health, that any transition between one level of care and another is fraught with peril. As a patient and family progress in a level of care, movement to a less restrictive level of care indicates progress. One would expect that it would be a welcome development, but with progress comes letting go of the very treaters and relationships that have held the patient and family through a tumultuous time. The idea of moving to a new team, maybe to a different location, feels more like abandonment as it means letting go of something that has worked and a team that is trusted. Because of this, many treatment episodes end at a transition point, either touching the next level of care very briefly or never even making it to the next level of care.

We take any transition between one level of care and another seriously and often rethink the procedure so that it feels as fluid and relational as possible. The procedural part is the easier part. It involves anticipating an available bed or slot, executing the timely sharing of clinical information, and managing financial needs prior to any movement. But the relational part is more subjective and involves a significant emotional component. For this, we use what we call a "warm hand-off." In our organization, a warm hand-off means that the treating clinician must act as an ambassador for the patient and family as they approach a new level of care. The sending clinician reaches out and speaks directly to the accepting clinician in the new level of care. This is an in person often telephonic communication.

While we all rely on an electronic medical record to convey the data needed in each case, we rely on the hand-off to communicate the "color" or "tone" in the case, which is not in the written record. It is incumbent on the sending clinician to speak to the relationships that have been formed, identifying the challenges or pitfalls that may have occurred and how they were addressed and hopefully overcome. We ask our clinicians to be honest and transparent about problems which may have occurred in treatment (not to sugarcoat anything) as well as to "market" the case to best position it for success in the next level of care. Importantly, once this is complete, the sending clinician must inform the patient and family about the interaction. We want the family to have the receiving clinician's name and to know that the receiving clinician is well informed of their needs and eager to work with them. We have found that absent this personal piece in a transition, a receiving program and clinician will inevitably focus on what may not have worked well and anticipate failure.

Case example: Changes in level of care

An exasperated mother asked to speak with a program administrator and when he returned her call, he politely asked what her concern was. "I'm afraid my daughter will die" was the response. She talked about her concern that her daughter, age 26, was being discharged from the acute care unit to a partial hospitalization program. The mother was convinced that her daughter was not yet ready for the change in level of care and again shared her overwhelming concern for her daughter's well-being.

The program administrator spoke with the treatment team and learned that the step down was not precipitous but part of a reasonable plan to help the young patient assume more responsibility and control over her treatment. Moreover, the team felt that the time spent on the inpatient unit had been productive and that the young woman had indeed turned a corner. She was doing better, citing several recent changes. Unfortunately, for the mother, the inpatient unit represented safety for her, and her family and she felt that any movement would be a real loss. She talked about experiencing great relief knowing that her daughter was safe in the hospital and well cared for. For this mother, any change to that arrangement felt frightening and full of risk. She struggled with the possibility that her daughter would again slide into her illness.

Although the mother had been educated about movement in the system when her daughter was admitted, she couldn't recall some of the important points of that discussion during this time of stress. The team decided to slow down the transition and to meet with the family face to face to again review the organization's philosophy about the levels of care in their system and most importantly, to stress an assurance that the system would stay with the family even if things seemed not to be working out. It was felt that this mother needed to hear that her concerns were legitimate and while shared by the team were mitigated by their confidence that the partial hospital could still provide daily monitoring, like the hospital. The team assured the mother that if things started to veer off track, she was not alone. There were many eyes on her daughter, and if needed, a step up back to an inpatient level of care, even for a brief period, was an option.

C Discharge

The third transition point we will focus on is the point of discharge for a patient and their family. A discharge can occur either at the end of a treatment episode or at a transition from one program or level of care to another. In both cases, it is a stress-filled time and feels like an ending to the patient and family. The point of discharge serves as an opportunity to check the fluidity of our internal systems as well as to hear directly from the patient and family their perceptions of their treatment experience.

We look first at the mechanics of each discharge; did the steps leading up to the discharge happen as they were intended? Was the move to a next step in treatment appropriate for the clinical presentation and was information clearly communicated to the patient and family? Did the family feel adequately oriented to their next treatment experience and was communication, either written or verbal, sent in advance by the receiving outpatient?

Like many treatment systems, we also use a survey tool to solicit our patients' and families' perceptions of their treatment experience. Efforts are made to hand deliver the survey to each patient prior to their transition and we strive to get a high completion rate. The content of the survey is designed to gather information on each component of treatment ("I worked well with my clinician" or "The group program helped me progress in treatment"), with the wording designed to solicit how the patient "feels" about their time with us. We have found that asking about "feelings" is much more productive as it allows the patient and family to consider their treatment experience in its entirety and the gamut of feelings they may have experienced throughout. As with many surveys, we ask what we can improve on and importantly for our staff, we ask for the names of any staff members who have contributed in a positive way to their recovery journey. Importantly, the monthly results of the survey are shared with all program staff.

Making a system perform well in each domain requires extensive training, diligent implementation, and steadfast monitoring of each operational practice. While all leadership has a role in the monitoring and responding to these transition points and managing corrections when needed, the weight of that responsibility often falls to the Chief Operating Officer (COO). In our experience, it is this person who sets the standard for monitoring performance and is tasked in real time with responding when things are not working as they should. To get the job done, the COO must be detail oriented and manage in a direct and respectful manner. He or she must be comfortable being the tie breaker in a potentially contentious debate and able to make a quick decision. They must have the focus to follow through when an adjustment to the system is required without the need for consensus. And a good COO is a strong systems thinker, meaning that when there is a breakdown in the system, it is seen as a systems problem rather than the fault of an errant employee.

Case example: Managing patient flow in a system of care

We heard early in the development of our system that a few patients in our acute care service were leaving our system to go to the next level of care run by a competitor. Frankly, we were surprised and while it was difficult to determine when this would happen due to the volume of discharges each day, the why part of the question was more troubling. We began asking clinicians to report to the treatment team the discharge or transition plan for each patient on the day of discharge. We learned a lot when we were able to hear in real time where someone was going and most importantly created an opportunity to discuss why a discharge may have been planned for another system of care seemingly with the support of our own treatment teams.

While some clinicians reported the reason for the move to another system as a point of family preference (something that we would always honor), others were vague stating things like "the patient feels more comfortable with X provider because of the information she received from a friend." Attempts to question this and even push for a clearer understanding were at times challenged by our own clinicians.

With a closer look, we learned that these were invariably clinicians who conceptually failed to buy into the idea of a working system. In fact, they still preferred to see treatment as movement between independent providers and often looked for providers that they knew outside of our system to cover a specific treatment need. Predictably, their preferences often encouraged directing business in one direction with the promise certainly of good treatment but always with some return professional benefit, like referrals back to the clinician's private outpatient practice.

Correcting the problem required a clear and direct message from the COO. She insisted that discharges from one level of care in the system were to be made to other levels of care in the system except in cases of family preference. More importantly, she met individually with the wayward clinicians and insisted that they decide about whether they could buy into our concept that treatment woven together within a singular system is far superior to the fragmented approach of shopping for care in independent stores. She insisted that going forward, any patient needing continuing care in another level of care should not leave our system for reasons other than family or patient preference, and if this was to occur, a discussion directly with her was required.

References

Allcom, S. (Winter 1990). Using matrix organization to manage health care delivery organizations. *Hospital & Health Services Administration*, 35(4), 575–590.

Burns, L. R. (1989). Matrix management in hospitals: Testing theories of matrix structure and development. *Administrative Science Quarterly*, 34(3), 349+.

Essex, R., Kennedy, J., Miller, D., and Jameson, J. (2023). A scoping review exploring the impact and negotiation of hierarchy in healthcare organizations. *Nursing Inquiry*, 30, e12571. https://doi.org/10.1111/nin.12571

Evans, J. M., Commisso, E., Grudniewicz, A., Im, J., Veillard, J., and Richards, G. (2024) Managing the performance of healthcare networks: a 'dance' between control and collaboration. *Public Management Review*, 26(7), 2144–2168, DOI:10.1080/14719037.2023.2264873

Provan, K. G., Nakama, L., Veazie, M.A., Teufel-Shone, N.I., and Huddleston, C. (2003). Building community capacity around chronic disease services through a collaborative interorganizational network. *Health Education & Behavior*, 42, 646–662.

3

OBJECTIVES OF A BEHAVIORAL HEALTH SYSTEM OF CARE AND ITS COMPONENTS

Access to a system of care, focused treatment, and the ability to vary the intensity of services are the hallmarks of a well-functioning system of care. Together, they form the groundwork for what we refer to as a rational road to recovery; each makes logical sense to those entering and moving through the system, and if executed well, will result in an effective treatment experience. The case for developing systemic, coordinated approaches to care has been made previously in relation to larger systems (Stroul and Friedman 1986; Hogan 2003; Hodges et al. 2012) as well as specific clinical populations (Minkoff and Cline 2004; Katon and Unutzer 2006) while others have focused on the need for implementing evidence-based practices more broadly and effectively (Torrey et al. 2001; Kazdin 2008; Norcross et al. 2008). This chapter builds on and extends these ideas across levels of care.

The "rational road to recovery" is first experienced in the admission process. Admission into our system is a single admission, meaning that once you have entered the system, we know you and are committed to working with you throughout your treatment experience, however long that may take. Working with complicated mental health needs, it is essential to directly address and mitigate the negative experience many have felt before – the figurative "spin cycle" of rapid, unproductive admissions and discharges. Most families can report the experience of a degree of success in stabilization, followed by what feels like a precipitous discharge, and within a short period and with little external support begin to slide backward. We know from experience that this escalates a feeling of impending failure so with a phone call, we create access to a level of care

DOI: 10.4324/9781315177366-4

that meets the needs of the individual. If the need is for acute care, due to some escalation of behaviors, the receiving team can quickly address each and make a relatively brief intervention. To be able to anticipate that needs may arise and to know that one can quickly re-enter the system through an expedited admission process prevents many of these events from occurring. In short, it is important to normalize changes in need and to quickly provide access to episodic treatment through an expedited admission process.

This sense of commitment from the system of care connects a patient and family to the system in a real way and often greatly reduces everyone's anxiety. The nature of discussions of discharge or moving to another level of care can be seen in a different light as movement does not feel like stepping off a cliff with no way back. The commitment from the system if additional support is needed translates into "we have your back and want you to view our system as your family's resource. We are available when and if you need us."

Similarly, we want each patient and their family to experience continuity in treatment while in the system. The goal is to move a patient as seamlessly as possible from one level of care to another to meet their needs at any given time. For example, an individual who is struggling to maintain their personal safety in a low-intensity community-based level of care may need to move to a more acute and controlled level of care like inpatient or residential levels of care. These transfers between levels of care are all handled internally through our Admissions Team. It is their job to facilitate expedited access by prioritizing bed availability, communicating in real time with insurance providers, and sharing relevant clinical information with the program that is to receive the patient. Similarly, an individual who is now stabilized in an acute level of care need not languish in an acute care bed until an appropriate slot in an outpatient program opens. Patients within our system are prioritized ahead of people seeking treatment from outside the system and can quickly move into less structured programming. This fluidity of movement between levels of care creates increased momentum for recovery.

Levels of care

There is no rigid formula for a system of care in behavioral health, and no specific set of programs that must be present to be called a system. Many systems tend to have a similar array of components; for instance, most will have some form of an acute level of care with each system tailored by the organization for the anticipated needs of the population it is designed to serve. As programming has developed over years and as support for systems has grown, many current behavioral health systems include some combination of the following program levels:

Acute inpatient

Patients admitted to this level of care are at a crisis time in their illness and as such should meet criteria that demonstrate the need for twenty-four-hour nursing and medical care in a structured, and possibly locked, treatment setting. From a clinical standpoint, acute inpatient programs are designed to conduct a rapid assessment of the presenting problem, initiate a brief and focused treatment intervention, and provide discharge planning to an appropriate next level of care. Treatment is focused specifically on the presenting precipitant to the admission, with searching for underlying dynamics or long-term treatment needs discouraged. The primary goal of an acute inpatient unit is to address an individual's basic safety needs, disrupt any maladaptive behavior patterns, and move the individual back into their community. It is generally understood that an inpatient hospitalization will not completely resolve the presenting problem nor provide a comprehensive treatment for the illness as many acute care settings operate with the understanding that acute symptomatology is episodic and time limited, and that long-term treatment, which is essential, is best provided in the community.

From a payer's perspective, due to the high cost of this level of care, there is an ever-present pressure on the acute care staff to quickly create some change in the presenting presentation and to identify a "step down" to a less restrictive level of care as soon as possible. Many insurance companies require daily updates from the treatment team on progress, and when a complication is identified, there is an immediate request for a plan to resolve it. Treatment can feel rushed, and if a patient and family are not informed about how the system works, this can easily cause confusion and upset.

In addition to the pressures on an acute care setting for quick change and movement, there are often several forces working against even the best of services. From the perspective of the family and outpatient system, an acute setting can be perceived as a respite from an exhausting experience. Both have likely been immersed in a crisis for the days leading up to the admission and it is common for families and providers to retreat and need time to regroup once the patient is safe in an acute setting. It is not uncommon for a family and an outpatient team to distance themselves post crisis knowing that the individual is safe and out of harm's way. This can be shown as a slowdown in communication, or more drastically when a block or seemingly insurmountable problem emerges. For instance, some families might use the time that their loved one is in the hospital to reassess a living arrangement or to change the degree of support they were offering. They may announce to the acute care treatment team that they have decided that the individual cannot return to their home or current living arrangement. Similarly, outpatient teams may use this time to rethink their treatment commitment with some developing their own criteria that the patient must meet to return to their care. Some requests are modest, reasonable goals, like agreeing to resume structured meetings with an actionable safety plan, but some are more unrealistic and unattainable, like assuring that the patient will be free from the behaviors which originally brought them into treatment.

Given the challenges facing an acute care service, things can quickly start to feel like a two-tier service rather than a system of care. The result is a tendency to hold a patient in an acute care setting for longer than may be clinically needed rather than gambling on a safe discharge if there are limited or inadequate disposition options. These challenges are significantly reduced, however, in a functioning system of care as each level of care is available for exactly the purpose it was designed for. This translates into shorter lengths of stay in acute care and much easier access to community-based programs and providers. It is the mobility between and among programs that ensures that no one program will be overly burdened and left holding the patient unnecessarily. This works because individual providers and programs from within the system know that they have easy access to acute care when and where they truly need it. From both the payer and patient perspectives, these are huge benefits.

Staffing acute care settings bears special mention as it presents numerous challenges both in incorporating different behavioral health disciplines and in maintaining the energy and enthusiasm needed to run an acute care setting. Acute care settings can be exceedingly taxing on program staff, and as such, it is not unusual for turnover to be high. Many staff members from all disciplines work for a year or two and then start to think about moving onto some other setting or area. This was particularly evident during the pandemic where across the country acute care settings struggled to maintain onsite clinical and nursing staff. As with all employees, there was a high concern about contagion which seemed amplified with the allure of internet-based practices which were often run from home.

While there is never a sure fix for any of these challenges, we have concentrated our efforts in finding ways to recognize our inpatient talent and to work to retain those rare individuals who truly enjoy the activity and challenge of an acute setting. For these folks, there is a joining in the mission of the organization and the role that an acute care setting plays as well as a sense of camaraderie which develops in the day-to-day work. Program staff members develop a bond through the emotion of the work in which an unspoken commitment to each other and the work is created. These individuals tend to take great satisfaction in accepting patients and families into the program at the height of a crisis and then thoughtfully moving them forward to a less restrictive level of care. Additionally, many of our acute care staff members reported that even during the pandemic, they appreciated the opportunity to come to work and developed a sense of pride in their ability to sustain the program.

Acute residential treatment

Although some payers shy away from the idea of funding for "residential care," we find this level of care can play an important role in affording a patient the opportunity to take measured steps back into the community. Residential programs provide community treatment and are unlocked. They can often provide a longer length of treatment than more expensive hospital stays and provide a structured and supportive environment. Most residential programs rely on group-oriented treatment modalities and case managers who can plan the next step in care.

Historically, residential programming has proven useful in the treatment of several disorders, including adolescents struggling with a home or family problem and adult patients struggling with substance use. In both cases, this level of care provides additional time and support to maintain a level of stability. In general, while still regarded as an acute level service, these programs are less expensive to run than inpatient hospitals as they rely on fewer high-cost medical resources. For many individuals, they can provide clinical support and a practicing ground for the skills needed to safely move into the community. Additionally, some residential programming can provide a diversion option for direct inpatient admission, thereby potentially averting a more costly inpatient hospitalization.

Partial hospitalization programs

Also regarded as an acute level of care, Partial Hospitalization Programs are an important component of a behavioral health treatment continuum and have grown in popularity. These programs generally operate during the business day Monday through Friday and provide a level of service and structure that is like a day spent in a psychiatric hospital. The major difference between an acute care hospital bed and a Partial Hospital Program is that the patient in a partial hospitalization program is deemed safe enough to go home at the end of the day. This, of course, means that the patient must be stable enough to live outside of a locked setting. Services provided are designed to integrate the patient back into their community and for the most part mirror the intensive, high resource staffing pattern and programming of an acute inpatient unit. Importantly, due to the limited program time, there is obviously a much lower cost than a full bed day of an acute care unit.

For these reasons, Partial Hospitalization Programs have an appeal to both patients and payers. From the patient perspective, the program is normalizing and less stigmatizing. It affords the patient the opportunity to receive support while remaining connected to their home and family and any community contacts. For many, it can be a level of care that provides a doable transition from an acute care setting, and in many cases, access to an acute hospitalization should the need arise provides a backup. From a payer's perspective, a Partial Hospital Program is a win. With cost often half that of an inpatient day, it allows funding support often for longer lengths of time and most importantly keeps the patient engaged in their community rather than an institution.

In a system of care, Partial Hospital Programs are designed to support an individual in two ways. First, they can be used as a step down from acute care for someone who may need additional support to successfully transition into the community. And second, they serve as a "front door" diversion from a hospitalization. In this scenario, an admission into a Partial Program can be used to avert a more expensive acute hospitalization while simultaneously providing structure and a high degree of support.

A Partial Hospital used in this way can help reduce recidivism for patients who may often be in crisis and tend to seek out acute care treatment. Partial programs provide a real-time opportunity to use new strategies or skills where and when real-world stressors occur.

Throughout the pandemic, many existing partial hospitalization programs mobilized quickly and developed the capacity to deliver their service virtually. Their efforts were supported by regulators and payers. Although somewhat variable in terms of quality, many of these virtual programs have clearly excelled. They can provide a robust and highly professional service online with clear advantages in access. A virtual partial hospitalization program provides access to behavioral health populations anywhere who might otherwise have had to manage long daily commutes to a treatment center. They also serve individuals who might never have shown up for treatment at all due to a personal reluctance to approach a brick-and-mortar behavioral health institution. While virtual programming might not work for everyone, and while clearly in need of more research in terms of accessibility and treatment outcomes, for many, they have created a very important opportunity for treatment.

From a system's management perspective, Partial Hospital Programs can be a challenge. Though not as expensive in terms of staffing as a twenty-four-hour-a-day hospital program, partial programs do employ many of the same behavioral health disciplines and must be prepared to respond to a crisis when it arises. As such, it is an expensive level of care. To make it work from a business sense, it is incumbent on partial programs to maintain or exceed their budgeted census. This can create problems as even with the best of clinical interventions, patients in a Partial Program do tend to miss program days and at times stop attending altogether. As is the case in many healthcare settings, once a person begins to feel better, program adherence tends to decline. For an expensive program in which patients decide daily if they want to attend, this can be very challenging.

Intensive outpatient programs

Although initially developed to assist individuals struggling with a substance use disorder, this level of care has expanded to all behavioral health disorders. An Intensive Outpatient Program affords several extended program visits per week in an outpatient setting. Most programs combine both individual and group modalities and run for two to three hours per day with clients finding shared support, psychoeducation, skill building, and treatment monitoring. Like a Partial Hospital Program, clients can attend while living at home and maintaining some normal activities of daily life, including school and work

Many intensive outpatient programs also changed over the course of the pandemic to a virtual platform. While the impact of this change is unclear at present, it seems evident that online Intensive Outpatient Programs increased access by removing travel for certain groups and reducing the stigma often associated with seeking mental health treatment. A big advantage of online services is the high degree of anonymity participants can enjoy.

Outpatient treatment

Long regarded as the stalwart of all behavioral health treatments, outpatient therapy has changed dramatically over the past decade. The addition of higher intensity levels of care and increased management from payers has decreased the duration of outpatient treatment courses and altered the dynamic of treatment through the adoption of only certain evidence-based practices. No longer is therapy open ended and exploratory in nature. Payers today insist that treatments be evidence based and use protocols that can be monitored by the payer to ensure expected lengths of each treatment episode and effect. Additionally, almost all health insurers prioritize the development of their treatment networks and only contract with outpatient providers who agree to work within set parameters. As a result, almost all outpatient work is focused in its approach and consistent with established evidence-based treatments that target specific disorders.

Importantly, the pandemic has spurred significant growth of behavioral health utilization among all age groups and in that growth has seen a dramatic increase in individuals seeking outpatient therapy. With increased acceptance of virtual treatment platforms, much outpatient treatment today is provided virtually. Services can now be accessed in almost any location with specialized treaters more accessible. With many positives, there are some downsides. Providers and licensing entities continue to struggle with how to negotiate current licensing requirements to accommodate online treatment across state lines. Additionally, with the ever-increasing shift in behavioral health providers into private practice and away from brick-and-mortar treatment centers, attracting providers to onsite programs has proven increasingly difficult.

Home-based treatment interventions

Home-based interventions emerged during the 1990s and were bolstered by the success of some treatment models that showed promise working with clients in their own home. These interventions rely on creative teams of professionals and paraprofessionals who are available to meet with families or individual patients in their homes rather than the more traditional clinic office. Engaging with patients and families on their own turf is in many respects clinically brilliant. It certainly solves the treatment accessibility problem for individuals with limited transportation and can be accommodating to a patient or family in terms of scheduling. More important, however, is that this treatment is literally on a patient or family's own terms. The model changes the power dynamic of treatment and likely provides more clinical information about what was going on in an individual's life.

While home-based treatment is effective, it does present some challenges. The first is a reluctance on behalf of many providers to relinquish their office space, which usually means convenience and a certain degree of power or authority, and move treatment into someone's home. Many also express concerns for personal safety citing the unpredictability of some individuals and the risk of being in some neighborhoods. These models are also costly. They provide a good deal of downtime and require the added expense of transportation to and from a patient's home. From the payer's side, it has been difficult to develop rates that truly support the model and there are also challenges in monitoring treatment without the formal structure of a clinic office. Despite these concerns, many payers now support home-based models and even reimburse for travel time. In many states, child and adolescent models rely heavily on in-home support.

We expect that as current system models push the acceptance of community programming, and as payers for behavioral health services have become more confident in home-based treatment, that we will see an increase in these models of intervention. This is already evident in several states where community programming, even in the context of a psychiatric emergency, occurs through home- or community- based models.

Internet-based treatment interventions

As with all systems of care, specific program components are fluid, and we would expect that current programs will evolve, and new ones develop to meet the changing needs and expectations of patients and their families. In many respects, the only limit in development is in the creative thinking of provider organizations. An example of this is the increasing use of the internet for online behavioral health services, including telemedicine and easily accessed apps.

There is no question that the proliferation of internet use increased during the pandemic when demand and accessibility required the relaxation of state and national regulations. Post pandemic, with models in many levels of care, virtual programming and hybrid configurations have become commonplace. Despite current challenges to privacy concerns and limitations on the flexibility of licensure for behavioral health professionals across state lines, we expect resolution to these problems and a future that will see these services expand.

Additionally, internet-based apps that record patient data and can communicate in real time to a patient, clinician, or treatment team are currently emerging, with many showing preliminary data to support their efficacy. As systems of care evolve, we anticipate an increase in access to online services and the potential for new and innovative treatments too dynamic and accessible to ignore.

References

Hodges, S., Ferreira, K., and Israel, N. (2012). "If we're going to change things, it has to be systemic:" Systems change in children's mental health. *American Journal of Community Psychology*, 49(3–4), 526–537. https://doi.org/10.1007/s10464-012-9491-0

Hogan, M. F. (2003). New freedom commission report: The President's new freedom commission: Recommendations to transform mental health care in America. *Psychiatric Services*, 54(11), 1467–1474.

Katon, W. J. and Unutzer, J. (2006). Collaborative care models for depression: Tiem to move from evidence to practice. Archives of internal medicine. *Arch Intern Medicine*, 166(21), 2304–2306.

Kazdin, A. E. (2008). Evidence-based treatment and practice: New opportunities to bridge clinical research and practice, enhance the knowledge base, and improve patient care. *American Psychologist*, 63(3), 146–159.

Minkoff, K. and Cline, C. A. (2004). Changing the world: The design and implementation of comprehensive continuous integrated systems of care for individuals with co-occurring disorders. *The Psychiatric Clinics of North America*, 27(4), 727–743.

Norcross, J. C., Hogan, T. P., and Kcocher, G. P. (eds.) (2008). *Clinician's Guide to Evidence-based Practices: Mental Health and the Addictions*. Oxford University Press.

Stroul, B. and Friedman, R. (1986). *A System of Care for Severely Emotionally Disturbed Children and Youth*. Georgetown University Child Development Center National Technical Assistance Center for Children's Mental Health.

Torrey, W. C., Drake, R. E., Dixon, L., Burns, B. J., Flynn, L., Rush, A. J., Clark, R. E., and Klatzker, D. (2001). Implementing evidence-based practices for persons with severe mental illnesses. *Psychiatric Services*, 52(1), 45–50.

4

STAKEHOLDERS AND DESIGN CONSIDERATIONS IN DEVELOPING BEHAVIORAL HEALTH SYSTEMS OF CARE

The Behavioral Health System of Care involves a complex interplay of various stakeholders, each with distinct roles and interests who wield significant influence over service delivery, policy formulation, and patient outcomes. Investors, regulators, payers, and employees constitute key components of this ecosystem, influencing policies, practices, and outcomes in mental health and substance abuse services. Investors in healthcare encompass a broad spectrum, ranging from private equity firms to philanthropic foundations. Their investments drive innovation, research, and infrastructure development within several emerging sectors and are largely unstudied in terms of relative quality, access, and return on investment (Gondi and Song 2019). Regulatory bodies play a crucial role in ensuring compliance, quality assurance, and patient safety across behavioral health services.

Payers, including government programs and private insurers, dictate reimbursement policies, coverage criteria, and care management strategies in behavioral health. Medicaid expansion and parity laws mandate equitable coverage for mental health and substance abuse services (Kaiser Family Foundation 2021). And last, the workforce within behavioral health organizations comprises diverse roles, including psychiatrists, therapists, social workers, and administrative staff. Their collective efforts are pivotal in delivering evidence-based interventions, fostering therapeutic relationships, and promoting recovery (AHA 2022). Furthermore, ongoing training and support programs enhance staff resilience, competence, and job satisfaction, thereby improving retention rates and service continuity (SAMHSA 2020).

DOI: 10.4324/9781315177366-5

All Behavioral Health Systems of Care exist for one reason only: to provide safe and effective treatment along with any necessary support for individuals who live with one or more moderate to severe behavioral disorders. And importantly, all major design decisions in both construction and operation must emanate from this core definition. In construction and in operation, each component of this definition also provides several reference points for evaluation of the effectiveness of the system. In other words, this core definition has power. It is both an internal guiding principle and a way to evaluate the success of the specific system at any point in time.

As with many things in behavioral health, systems of care are complicated. In fact, they are perhaps the most complicated at the point of start-up, though significant challenges continue over time particularly as they grow. The initial challenge is all about system "architecture," how to get the basic building blocks, the key clinical programs, off the ground. Later, the challenges are often "processes," how to get the system to actually work well "as a system" where the parts collaborate in service of the patients and their families. Another issue at inception and at key moments along the way is that systems must work to configure themselves to the differing and sometimes conflictual needs of a variety of established stakeholders. These stakeholders may challenge some of the basic design assumptions and add desired outcomes different than the initial definition. But starting from the beginning, each system of care hits the ground with numerous stakeholders, each with an agenda, and some of which compete with one another. We identify these as investors, regulators, payers, employees, and of course, patients or clients.

Investors are the individuals who use their cash to fund the idea and building of the project. The idea of the system or a specific program within the system must be appealing to them first and foremost as an investment. This simply means that the investors who participate in the project expect that by investing their cash, they will get a return. And while there can be many types of investors, each will vary within two important expectations: the amount of return expected and timeline for that expected return. One thing that never seems to vary is the "risk" profile of these and other healthcare ventures where there is significant capital investment in facilities and talent. A great deal of cash is expended before the first dollar of reimbursement is ever collected. This is especially true when hospital level of care is involved.

In our experience, investing in a Behavioral Health System of Care is likely to be more successful than investing in single program or level of care organizations; however, many behavioral health organizations fail to make it to "system" status and achieve limited commercial success or suffer losses. One thing for sure: this is not the area to target for a quick return on investment. Systems need time to reach a level of maturity before they can generate healthy returns. And while behavioral health growth is generally slower than growth in other segments of healthcare, developing and growing a new system is often beset by unanticipated perils. Business plan projections that seem manageable at the outset of a project with an anticipated slow ramp-up and incremental growth are almost routinely disrupted by real-life events that interfere as the system is developing. A case in point occurred days before the opening of our new, long-awaited flagship, 82-bed facility at Walden Behavioral Care. A worker putting the final touches on the fire suppression system failed to secure a major pipe on the second floor. By the next morning, a small lake of foul water had flooded one end of the brand-new inpatient unit and the same on the floor beneath. Life happens. The facility opening was delayed more than two weeks and the remediation cost exceeded $100,000. Although the cost of the damage was eventually covered by contractor's insurance, there was limited reimbursement for the lost revenue and no reimbursement for the ripple effects of the delay like additional rent that had to be paid at the current facility.

Some investors are drawn to a behavioral health project for personal interest, perhaps their own experience with behavioral health needs or that of a family member. In these situations, they are "leading with their heart" but they are savvy businesspeople, too. Often, they are driven to improve things or to re-make a system so that it works better for people in need. Many come into these projects wanting the project to be distinct or innovative. They are convinced that it will add to the healthcare landscape in some way, and in addition to being successful against the other systems that it will compete with, believe it will ultimately enhance treatment. With some personal interest, they tend to have a singular vision of what they are supporting and strong opinions about how and when components should be developed. With their past financial success, they come to the table with a degree of confidence and have specific ideas about how the system may change the healthcare landscape with others more focused on the details of a system's operations. Regardless, all investors exert a degree of pressure on the development and implementation of a new or developing system.

The same is true, though for different reasons with state and federal regulators. These individuals, often employees of the state in which the programs are located, have significant leverage in the building or expanding of a system of care. Regulators provide the licensure or permissions needed for the system of care to open and once open, to continue to operate. They wield significant power, particularly in the implementation phase as programs ready to open. Whatever the project, it must line up with their established criteria in regulation for the project to gain approval and move forward. As they work only through regulations, they often struggle with innovation in programming.

Changes are often in conflict with established program specifications, and many regulators are not known for their flexibility. Efforts to adapt programming to regulation and waivers obtained for uncharted regulatory areas can take time and are best addressed as far ahead of time as possible. And once a program is open, regulators can return on an ongoing basis as enforcers. Here, they check to see that the now licensed program is adhering to their expectations. If not, program operations can be curtailed, and in some extreme circumstances, licenses revoked.

Case example

One excellent example in a system of care involved conflicting regulations and expectations regarding program participation in two levels of care, inpatient and residential, both acute care programs supervised by different branches of the same agency. In the planning phases, everyone agreed that a core value of the acute system was the active engagement of the patient group. It was envisioned that everyone in the programs would be involved in a robust group program and participate in a highly interactive therapeutic milieu. We came to learn that in the state in which they were located, there was a separate licensing entity for each. One state department licensed only acute care units and another state department, entirely different, regulated residential programs.

As expected, there were many common points between the two groups of regulators but also some significant differences. Where it really fell apart was around use of patient rooms. The residential licensing group strongly supported the value of an active milieu and as such supported a program expectation that once up in the morning, patients were to spend most of their day in common programs spaces with other patients and staff. Although no one would refuse a patient's wish to spend time in their room, there was a program expectation for active participation which the program leadership was hopeful could create a culture of a strong milieu. Unfortunately, the inpatient regulators had different expectations. For them, a patient's access to their room at any time was seen as a human right. They disagreed with any expectation that patients would spend most of their day outside of their rooms. For them, there was a strong value that each patient should have access to the privacy and comfort of their own space at any time. Despite best efforts, it became clear that there was no room for negotiation.

The result was that each program in the acute care part of the system had different expectations for patient participation. In the hospital, some patients who were not interested in joining the milieu elected to spend much or sometimes all their day in the privacy of their rooms. In the residential program, with the rule that all were expected to be out of their rooms, the opposite occurred. This was highlighted as a systemic problem when one mother complained that her daughter, who had recently been stepped up from the Residential Program, confessed to her that she liked the inpatient unit better. It was her perception that the inpatient unit was less restrictive than the residential program as in the inpatient unit she was allowed to spend the entire day in bed in her room. The mother was distressed at such different program expectations and that her daughter had found a way to remain on the inpatient unit and essentially stuck in her treatment.

Like regulators, payers of care hold great sway in the development and ongoing operation of a Behavioral Health System of Care. We saw this with the early interventions in the 1980s which came about mostly through private insurers and their clear need to contain ballooning behavioral health costs. Some private sector insurance companies were the first to use the power of the payer to creatively flex benefits designs that afforded funding for interventions that moved a patient away from a hospital and into the community. In essence, they were the pioneers who essentially designed and funded the first systems of care, though on a very small scale.

Payers

The power of the payer comes from the reality that each insurance company decides what services they want to have in their treatment network and how to structure a contract with each provider for services. A lot has changed since the early days as services are not individually crafted to address a need. Today, they are carefully prescribed through written performance specifications that assure consistency of programming across networks serving a state or even national geography. On one hand, this consistency has been a good thing; it has proved a blueprint for levels of care and assures a common understanding in the behavioral health community about each service and what must be provided. However, this uniformity does come at a cost. As past innovations have been integrated into the behavioral health landscape and accommodate larger populations, creating additional change or innovation becomes more complex. The result is that today there are fewer exceptions or changes.

Once the idea of innovation occurred in the private sector, public sector payers, specifically Medicaid, created large-scale systemic changes in the mid-1990s. Many states proposed waivers to Centers for Medicaid and Medicare Services and created demonstration projects aimed at containing costs certainly but also improving access and enhancing quality. Due to the volume of Medicaid members in each state, these innovations were coupled with a high volume of customers which fueled the development of different programs that would eventually create levels of care. Medicaid encouraged the use of dollars to creatively provide services in non-conventional settings and with programs outside of the bricks and mortar of hospitals. One example is the funding through Medicaid of Partial Hospitalization Programs. Once unheard of, these programs proliferated across the country and became an alternative to keeping individuals in locked hospitals by giving them a community-based program with the clinical support of a hospital.

When a new system of care is developing, part of the process is to identify the larger groups of individuals who will seek out those services and proactively solicit payers who will send their members in need to those services. Although it is hard to move large systems, there is often room for some creativity given enough lead time and the ability to demonstrate cost savings.

As a result, each individual system is looking for multiple outcomes, financial returns for investors, job satisfaction and benefit structure for employees, and of course, treatment experience and outcome for the recipient of the service. Common to all these systems is that each of these "customers" has an investment in the system having paid into it in some way. And perhaps most important is that the people paying into the system want a voice. We'll cover this in more depth later, but suffice it to say, that when additional layers of expectation are added to the core purpose of the system, the focus can easily shift, wander, or at times, get completely lost. In practice, this shows a remarkable lack of coordination, something that is more often the rule than the exception.

We talked about the contribution of investors, regulators, and payers, but by far the greatest consideration in planning and operating a system of care are the people, both employees who staff all programs and the patients or clients that attend programs looking for treatment. Both groups are stakeholders in the truest sense of the word but surprisingly often overlooked in planning. In this discussion, we will consider each group separately: the people who work in the system (administrators, support staff, clinicians) and the people who the system serves (the patients or clients).

Employees

We don't usually think about the people who work in the system as "design elements," but there is a lot to say for recruiting and populating the endeavor with people who understand and are committed to the core definition or purpose of Behavioral Health System of Care. If this can be done early in the system's development, they can be a powerful asset in creating the culture as a group working toward a common goal. We acknowledge that all contributors are important, and we speak a lot throughout this book about the critical role that leadership or administrators play in a system and similarly recognize the power that support staff play in establishing and carrying an organizational culture. All are important. While good architecture and strong processes are necessary, having the people who show up every day with the right attitude and a willingness to "buy-in" to providing care in a prescribed manner is what really determines whether the system functions as it is intended.

But not all employee groups provide the same challenges. We have found that it is the clinician group, regardless of specific discipline, that presents the greatest challenge in creating a sense of "buy-in" and truly investing in a system of care. This might seem surprising as one would think that there would be many good reasons for professionals to "buy-in," but in truth, this is not a given. Clinicians vary widely in preferences for whom they want to work with and even within that, how and where they want to work. For instance, some clinicians prefer to work with patients over a long course of an illness while others don't have the same "drive" to manage treatment over time and will resist long-term clients. Some clinicians feel much more competent working with short-term treatment models and need near-term, tangible results in their work. Additionally, many clinicians seem distrustful of the work of others. They've been trained to practice in relative isolation with limited real understanding of the work of their peers and resist being monitored or rated for their work. And last, almost all clinicians vary in how they think about the process of change and recovery having been oriented in their training to a certain philosophy that may not be embedded in a particular system of care. For them, agreeing to follow a specific treatment model and an accompanying program philosophy may feel foreign and ultimately not a good fit for a particular system. If that's the case, especially after sufficient training that explains and describes the Behavioral Health System of Care and the ways in which individuals are expected to participate, it is better to part ways. No harm, no foul – it's not for everybody.

But what are the reasons for a clinician to "buy-in" and invest in a system of care? They are numerous and they are profound.

1 People who work in behavioral health do so with a commitment to provide relief and healing to the people they serve. A well-conceived Behavioral Health System of Care operates from the same set of basic human values that attracted these individuals to the field in the first place. In most of the programs we're worked in, we are open with our belief that people do this work for deeply personal reasons. It's important to know that the reason may not be entirely conscious to a person as they begin this work and it may, in fact, change over time, but it is there. We create a time usually in a staff meeting and will pose the question "what is it about this work that draws you to it?" What usually follows is a powerful telling of reasons that people have for committing to the work they do, and for some, this may be the first time that they fully articulate the reasons for choosing this career. Even more powerful is the realization and then the esprit de corps that emerges when

the individual appreciates that they are surrounded by other individuals who share in this commitment.

2 The work of providing treatment to individuals with significant behavioral disorders can be quite difficult on an emotional basis for the treater who feels the burden of the patients' distress and strives to make a difference in their lives. A well-conceived behavioral health system of care works to take the burden off the individual and to make it into a "team sport," where accountability and responsibility are shared not only with the multidisciplinary treatment team within the program but across the expanse of the system. Care in this sense is owned "by the system" with the knowledge that adjacent programs can continue the work that has begun in another program. No individual is expected to carry the physical and emotional load of attaining a "cure" by themselves and this greatly lessens the possibility that a treating clinician will "take the work home with them," a major source of staff burnout.
3 Because a well-conceived behavioral health system shares the treatment course among a group of related programs, the result is that the focus of treatment is often better defined. With this understanding, the internal components of treatment are more specifically designed to achieve certain outcomes that define specific successes for a program or a phase of treatment. Over time, individuals and teams working in these environments come to understand their roles better, become more expert in the aspect of care they provide, and build experience with the treatment population. This leads to a higher sense of mastery for the program and team. For individuals engaged in these endeavors, having the sense that one is doing a good job and contributing to the greater systemic good is immensely satisfying. This is a vast improvement over other behavioral health treatment environments in which clinicians have overly broad responsibility and don't have the advantage of clarity about what is expected from them.

Patients or clients

Without question, considering the needs of the individuals who will use the system is perhaps the greatest area of consideration in planning and development of the system. In fact, if the system fails to meet the clinical needs of individuals seeking service within it, it will undoubtedly fail as a treatment entity and as a business. We strongly encourage including the perspective and voice of the consumer in the planning and ongoing operation of a system of care.

Fortunately, the paradigm of how we understand people with lived experience has shifted dramatically over the years. While our language has improved, it is essential that as system planners, we design with the end user in mind and ask for input in every facet of development. This requires that we really work to include consumers in the process and listen carefully to what is offered. There are opportunities to include these individuals in planning committees, oversight boards, and ethics committees as well as in the operations of the system as employees. We have learned that whatever avenue is used for inclusion, it should be done transparently and with the full support of senior management. The organization will reap numerous benefits from this practice, including better facility and program design decisions as well as a more sophisticated employee attitude that comes from working alongside recovered consumers.

Design elements

Given all of this, it may be a bit of a surprise, but the reality is that it may well be easier to build a well-functioning Behavioral Health System of Care from the ground up than to take an existing (and most likely a failing system) and attempt to fix it. A new system has no negative history to overcome and begins as a clear idea with specific values that become a well thought out blueprint. That concept can, over time, grow into several programs, some of which work with remarkable coordination. A system that begins from such an elegant inception has the advantage of foresight and direction (even if this changes over time). Most important, however, is that this path often begins with motivated and visionary leadership: individuals who can "see" the completed system and can enthusiastically communicate that to investors and program staff. Part of that communication is a pioneering or innovative drive that infuses the organization with excitement and energy.

Case example

Walden Behavioral Care began with a phone call from a Commissioner of Mental Health who was looking to save an inpatient psychiatric unit that was slated to close with the transition of a small community hospital to a community health center. The Commissioner knew that losing the inpatient unit, although small, would mean another loss of valued inpatient beds in a state that was working hard to maintain a viable private sector behavioral health service system. Additionally, this unit had developed into somewhat of a specialty service in eating disorders, an illness that at the time was under the radar of most providers and for which few services even existed. Her call was timely and directed toward the right people. A transition plan was developed and a vision for the service set. Most of the program staff, eager to maintain their employment, responded to the idea of growing the unit into a strong behavioral health presence and expressed a willingness to work to enhance the specialty service of eating disorders.

Though not entirely a new program, the re-starting of a service slated to close provided the right mix of need and enthusiasm. Existing staff members re-invested in the service and quickly bought into the vision of the new leadership. Within months, a new program was opened, and a system of care was born.

Importantly, many systems of care are built onto existing systems and importantly share a similar focus and organizational culture. The major design elements within Behavioral Health System of Care are generally thought of as the following three elements: programs and services to be or already being delivered, the processes that exist within and between these "subsystems," and the people who work in them. Let's look at these separately.

Programs or subsystems can be of almost any size. Some are quite small, for instance a select number of simple group structures formed to address a specific problem. These smaller systems engage a few dedicated individuals who tend to know each other professionally and importantly share a vision of the work the system is designed to accomplish. They tend to serve a small number of individuals across a limited geography. Other programs or subsystems can be more complex. They are usually populated by people from several professionals from a variety of disciplines, almost all of whom work independently of each other. These larger systems function as a whole and strive to deliver services on some routine basis and often across a larger geography.

With both scenarios, the systems may vary in terms of history. Some may have been around since behavioral health departed from the two-tier beginnings of a hospital-outpatient dyad, growing over time in level of care sophistication. And others are either more recently formed to address the changing landscape of behavioral health or are forming as we speak, fueled by a good idea and supported by a market analysis. They are usually funded by a willing commercial enterprise which can supply the financial resources to bring it to life.

Regardless, the processes of a Behavioral Health System of Care regardless of size are critical to any successful operation. When a system is working well, it is because the necessary processes are in place and are working as they are intended. We describe this as "the whole is greater than the sum of the parts." This means that the impact on and the ultimate success on users of the System is greater than if similar services were acquired or sequenced independently. This is the "magic" of a system, and it creates an enhanced effect when the programs or subsystems within the system utilize organizational processes in similar ways. They work in synchronicity. Specifically, each program or service and each staff member in the organization views themselves as part of a complex holistic treatment effort. It is then that a system can provide healing as intended.

The role of program definition in system design

We think of movement in a system of care as one of the core features needed to keep treatment in each level of care true to its specific definition and for a patient to feel a sense of momentum and progression (even if the movement is back to a more intensive level of care). But maintaining program flow, the actual moving of patients from one level of care to another as soon as possible, is difficult. There is a tendency in a system of care for each program level to take on more than its prescribed contribution to the smooth operation and achievement of positive clinical outcomes. This happens for a few reasons, including the comfort and familiarity of the patient and family in a specific program or to a group of staff members, as well as a natural hesitancy to accept someone new into a receiving program. In the service of keeping patient flow operating, it is essential that there be a clear definition of what each component is to accomplish in a case and specifically its role in the greater system.

In establishing this definition, it's also important for the program to have a good understanding of what is not included in the definition. A clear example of role definition in a Behavioral Health System of Care is the generally acknowledged purpose of psychiatric inpatient or hospital programs. All would agree that the function of these programs is the medical and psychiatric stabilization needed in any given case. Individuals are often hospitalized for safety purposes with the goal of disrupting the unsafe behaviors and establishing some understanding of why they are occurring (although achieving this can be a complex task). A patient in an acute care hospital is not there to receive in-depth psychotherapy or achieve therapeutic goals beyond the ability to maintain safety following their stay on an inpatient unit.

Once this definition is established, clinical leaders within the program can develop a course of treatment and implement the needed program components that can target the stated goal and establish criteria for discharge. One of the most positive things about this is that the performance of a program can be evaluated based on this definition, which affords improvements in programming and staffing when necessary. Such clarity of purpose and the focus that an accurate definition provides can lead to continued program improvement and ultimately patient success over time. Conversely, when program definition is diffuse, it is virtually impossible to evaluate the performance of programs, subsystems, and even staff members. What tends to happen on the patient's side is that due to the highly complex behavioral symptoms and life issues, patients become stuck. They can languish in a specific program or level of care often requiring sustained treatment that goes beyond the capability of any single program. The staff members and programs that try to treat them eventually default to an impossible though well-intended urge to "cure" the patient and this mostly results in sloppy treatment and chaos.

Perhaps the most important contributing factor in the clarity of program definition is the existence of another program/subsystem or group of programs that acts as a referral or "step down" (or step up). When interim clinical goals (i.e. stabilization in the case of inpatient programs) have been achieved for patients in the first program, having a place to go creates a dynamic of movement that allows each program to feel successful in fulfilling their role and the patient achieves a sense of progress in treatment. Additionally, having a good sense of individual program definition is enhanced by working cooperatively with one or more other programs that "pick up" the patient for the next phase of treatment. This is especially true when there is a "grand design" envisioned by leadership of the system which identifies core philosophical similarities, complementary features of the two programs, and the ways in which treatment continuity is intended to work. In other words, not only does one program take referrals from the other, but they are specifically designed to take referrals from each other routinely and to continue the achievements from one program within a similar framework that is transparent and understandable to the patient. When this occurs, transition from one program to the other is planned and predictable and results in far less stress and anxiety for all involved.

Interaction among programs in Behavioral Health System of Care

The way that programs within a Behavioral Health System of Care relate to each other determines the effectiveness of the System overall, and we regard the most important aspect of this as the "flow" or ease of movement between programs. The general idea is that patients move from program to program as their condition improves. We call this "stepping down," essentially progress in the right direction. There is significant value to patients when the System operates in a way to maximize the fit between a patient's needs and the program's capabilities. Importantly, Behavioral Health Systems of Care exist for the purpose of assisting individuals with major disorders of thought, mood, and behavior; the course of recovery is often not linear. Sometimes, patients need to step up, and sometimes, they can step down at a more accelerated pace, skipping some programs in between. While a system can be depicted as a flight of stairs, it is important to remember that all paths up or down the stairs are not equal. A treatment course is never set, but rather responsive to the changing needs of the patient and family. The ease of which a group of programs accommodate the patient's changing needs is a major way in which the System acts to individualize treatment. While this may sound easy, it's quite difficult to achieve, especially when the System is functioning at near or full capacity as has been the case with our primary example, Walden Behavioral Care. We will discuss this further in Chapter 5.

References

American Hospital Association (AHA). (2022). Strengthening the Healthcare Workforce. www.aha.org/system/files/media/file/2022/09/Strengthening-the-Health-Care-Workforce-Complete-20220909.pdf

Gondi, S. and Song, Z. (2019). Potential implications of private equity investments in health care delivery. *JAMA*, 321(11), 1047–1048.

Kaiser Family Foundation. (2021). Amid Unwinding of Pandemic-Era Policies, Medicaid Programs Continue to Focus on Delivery Systems, Benefits, and Reimbursement Rates: Results from an Annual Medicaid Budget Survey for State Fiscal Years 2023 and 2024. www.kff.org/report-section/50-state-medicaid-budget-survey-fy-2023-2024-introduction/

Substance Abuse and Mental Health Services Administration (SAMHSA). (2020). Workforce Development in Behavioral Health. www.samhsa.gov/sites/default/files/workforce-development-in-behavioral-health.pdf

5

HOW DOES A BEHAVIORAL HEALTH SYSTEM OF CARE WORK?

Building on several core concepts of systems of care, it's important to highlight the design and operational features that enable theoretical ideas to take effect in real-world situations. Others have written about the need for effective step-down programs that bridge the gap between inpatient and standard once weekly outpatient care (Mee-Lee et al. 2001; SAMHSA 2016) and the need for programming that varies in intensity as patients progress and sometimes regress during an episode of care (Davidson et al. 2005).

This chapter incorporates ideas that promote practices designed to enhance treatment effectiveness within specific programs such as the use of evidence-based practices and integrated care models (Torrey et al. 2001; Drake et al. 2005) and the use of specific interventions tailored to individual needs. This flexibility of approach is especially important in situations where there is a high degree of complexity of the population being treated (Torrey et al. 2001; SAMHSA 2016).

Additionally, organizational culture within behavioral health organizations plays a crucial role in the delivery of care. Collaboration among programs and between caregivers in the same program is key to providing a comprehensive, integrated treatment experience. According to Schein (2010), a culture that fosters collaboration, continuous learning, and adaptation to the needs of the population served can enhance the effectiveness of treatment services. Others have noted that a positive organizational culture is instrumental in implementing changes in existing mental health programs that lead to improved patient outcomes, including the integration of services, focus on recovery-oriented care, and the promotion of an inclusive environment for both staff and those receiving services (Mee-Lee et al. 2001; Aarons et al. 2011).

DOI: 10.4324/9781315177366-6

On the surface, it may appear that a Behavioral Health System of Care would operate similarly to other healthcare services. After all, there are many of them, and each appears to have some common systemic components and operating principles running in the background. It's what keeps our health system humming. But Behavioral Health Systems of Care are different from the rest. They require a set of expectations regarding communication and a set of "governing" rules that are ingrained into the organization and woven into the operations of the system. These expectations ensure that collaboration among the sub-parts is maintained in service to treatment continuity and patient satisfaction. In this chapter, we will describe the general operations of a Behavioral Health System of Care with the expectations and rules of each.

General operations of a Behavioral Health System of Care

Admissions: First contact and entry

A colleague called me at work upset and embarrassed. She told me that the night before her daughter had become so distraught that she felt she had to be admitted to a psychiatric hospital. My colleague doesn't work in behavioral health, but she does work in healthcare and honestly is an astute woman. Her problem she said, somewhat sheepishly, was that she had no idea how to go about accessing inpatient care. So, she told me that the night before she did what made sense. She and her husband loaded their escalated adolescent into the family car and drove to a neighboring town where she knew there was a private psychiatric hospital. Arriving in the dark of night and driving down a long drive toward the hospital, she said they felt disoriented. There was no sign of an entry point for new arrivals nor any well-lit buildings to orient to. They ultimately parked the car, and with her daughter in tow, walked up to the front door and knocked.

Their daughter was not admitted. Whoever answered the door seemed incredulous when they heard why they were there, and the family was unceremoniously told that this is not how it's done. I think she called me to reality check herself. Did she do something wrong? But then came the all too familiar exasperation at those of us in mental health who build and frankly tolerate such confusion. In her family's moment of need, we failed. They couldn't even find the front door to access care.

Long considered the unsung hero of most Behavioral Health Systems is the Admissions Department. Some might perceive this as a side function in an organization, almost lowly, but we would put it front and center. It is the hub of a bicycle wheel, the center point to accessing any system. It is also how many critical components of a system can be tracked and managed.

First contact with a Behavioral Health System of Care is almost always a phone call or electronic request for some sort of service. Inquiries come directly from patients or families, although sometimes from referring clinicians or other healthcare institutions (particularly if the request is for admission to or transfer from a medical hospital setting). The most efficient and customer friendly way for a Behavioral Health System of Care to manage these requests is through a community-facing clinical and administrative function variously referred to as "intake" or "access." Whatever term is used, it connotes entry to the larger body of services that are provided by the organization. For many reasons, the importance of the Admissions Department to the system of care cannot be overstated. It has four primary roles:

- To provide an easy and accommodating front door and first contact with new patients
- To gather clinical information and to provide a clinical assessment which in turn enables an efficient clinical triage
- To collect and verify insurance or reimbursement information to assure payment for services and utilization review
- To serve as the "air-traffic" control for the Behavioral Health System of Care as a whole, keeping tabs on the availability of services and patient flow or movement throughout the System

Given their importance, we consider each function separately.

To provide an easy and accommodating front door and first contact with new patients

While each of these functions of the Admissions Department is critical, the point of first contact with a patient and their family is certainly the most important to the consumers of services. Individuals seeking assistance with significant behavioral disorders are often in a compromised condition when they reach out and have likely been subjected to stigma related to their mental health in past dealings with other agencies and healthcare providers. They are inevitably frustrated, and all feel desperate for some form of relief. Because of this, the communication that occurs at the point of first contact with the system is pivotal. It is a likely determinant of whether an individual follows through in getting the help that they need and in many respects the success or failure of any treatment intervention.

We consider the function of admitting into the system as the hub of the operation. This means that all programs and services start and flow from this service. The Admissions Department is much more than a simple transfer of information, something that is especially true in a Behavioral Health System of Care where so much depends on the accurate gathering and conveying of information. Admissions professionals should be knowledgeable about the services the organization provides, patient, and friendly. They should be able to quickly create connection with the individual seeking service, make a critical triage decision based on the information they are given and then connect the client to the correct people or programs in the organization to advance the request for help.

All too frequently, organizations delegate admissions work to a clerical function and put people in these roles who are poorly trained, overburdened, and abrupt. Not only does this limit the actual admission, but it creates a negative perception of the entire institution and a poor start to treatment. It is essential that the entire admissions process be done well, from answering the first phone call and creating a sense of reassurance, to the clinical decision-making and ultimately to accessing the next steps in the process of getting treatment services.

To gather clinical information and to provide an assessment which in turn enables efficient clinical triage

The Admissions Department is where the patient record is "born," and today, this is almost always in an electronic format. Elements are entered that become the basic means in which patients are identified, clinically evaluated, and then advocated for both in terms of services to be rendered and methods of payment for services. If any information is inaccurate at the outset, the patient runs the risk of being denied treatment, referred to the wrong services, and/or being billed by the organization for services that are expected to be reimbursed by insurance providers whether public or private.

It may sound simple, but even something as basic as a name can cause confusion. In our work, we treat a high number of LGBTQ+ individuals. Many have chosen names that differ from the name registered with their health insurance carrier. Failure to capture the correct name on the insurance policy greatly increases the likelihood that coverage will be denied and conversely failure to use an individual's chosen name can be taken as an offense. So, it is important to ask for the name on their insurance policy and then to use and communicate with any treater who may interact with the patient the name the patient prefers.

Aside from basic demographic information, the process of connecting patients with the best services available starts immediately. Critical data exchanged during this time should include age of the patient as there is almost always a different set of services for youth and adults and some general idea of what problems or symptoms are presently active and what services the patient (and family) is seeking. This information does not have to be in depth but must be accurate as frequently the information from the initial contact will serve as a guide to routing the patient to the next point in the process, the clinical evaluation or triage.

The clinical evaluation provided by the Admissions Department is usually a structured interview that involves a more extensive discussion about the current and historic nature of the patient's difficulty and why they are seeking treatment at this time. It is the beginning of the clinical formulation that will inevitably guide this episode of treatment. It is also a time to gauge what the patient is looking for in terms of level of care and to assess whether this is realistic. This can be challenging as most patients come into a behavioral health system with an opinion, however formed, of what services they believe they need. Admissions staff members need to be able to hear what a patient would like and carefully and realistically balance that with their level of care criteria.

We have always used individuals with professional clinical credentials and training in our Admissions Department. They must be skillful in engaging the client and assessing the patient's actual symptom presentation and motivation or willingness to engage in treatment at this time. We use one or more standardized tests to assess patient functioning or symptom severity. This can assist the practitioner in making a determination about the level of care. Data such as this also provides a metric that is often useful to payers. And as an organization, the use of standardized testing and measurement over time provides a benchmark against which to measure progress in treatment. It is important however to note that the clinical evaluation is much more than an exchange of information. It can truly be thought of as the first step in treatment. We rely on the clinician to educate the patient in how the system works and setting realistic expectations for treatment in the therapeutic environment.

Clinical need refers to the condition of specific patients and providing them access to the level of care that is best suited to their situation at any point in time. Perhaps most critical in a Behavioral Health System of Care with an inpatient setting is gaining admission for a patient in severe distress to this level of care. Given the concern about a particular patient's condition, there are often numerous individuals, including family members, outpatient treatment professionals, public agency representatives, emergency rooms, etc. that are clamoring for an admission to take place as soon as possible. It could also be that a particular patient is already in the system but now requires a higher level of care, a common occurrence in systems that treat complex presentations.

Through all, the Admissions Department monitors program capacity, a concept that refers not only to the space available in a particular program but also the perceived ability of the program staff to treat the patient and the complexity of their specific condition. This perception of staff could be related to some novel issues presented by a particular patient or just the capacity of the program to provide care to the patient due to the presence of other complex patients in the program. In other words, the totality of the needs of the patient population at any given point in time needs to be considered. When staff experience a mismatch between patient need or population need and their capacity, they may resist placement of a particular patient in the program. When this occurs, higher level clinical leaders and administrators must step in to determine what to do next.

To collect and verify insurance or reimbursement information which assures payment for services and utilization review

The Admissions Department is also responsible for capturing specific data during the assessment needed to determine payment of services. This function is important to both the patient and the service provider and there may be numerous activities and considerations involved in determining the answers to key questions like "what services is the patient eligible for." Therefore, getting accurate data about the patient and their insurance coverage, if applicable, from the point of first contact is crucial. Without accurate data, services can easily be denied or go unpaid for long periods of time, requiring both the patient and provider to make time-consuming corrections later in the process, perhaps even after services have ended.

Critical to this process is establishing eligibility and especially with services at higher levels of care (hospital and residential), attaining prior approval from the payer. Insurance eligibility defines what services are available under a specific health plan. Each plan is governed by a specific document or contract between the patient and the insurer and can usually be checked or confirmed through an electronic database or by calling a representative of the insurer. Organizations that do not perform this function well do so at great peril as invoices for treatment services will be rejected and go unpaid unless and until eligibility can be established.

In this age when almost all healthcare is carefully managed by insurance companies, many services are subject to review by the insurer before they are approved. This practice is seen by insurers as a safeguard around overuse or overreliance on certain types of services, usually focused on utilization of inpatient or residential programming. The process can take multiple steps and can be appealed if the service request is rejected initially. Direct communication between senior clinical staff at the provider site and clinical staff at the insurer may be necessary to clarify the need and advocate for the patient on a case-by-case basis.

As insurance status can change on an almost daily basis, we have found it prudent to have our Admissions Department verify the status of each patient's insurance (often daily), and to carefully manage the communication between the service level and the utilization reviewer at the insurance company. Although we have experimented with several models, the most efficient has been to include the behavioral health system's *utilization management* team as part of the Admission Department. This affords our team ready access to current insurance data and allows us to capitalize on the relationships, some built over the years, with employees from our high-volume payers. These relationships, which we strive to craft as partnerships, rely on honesty. We practice clear and direct communication with a high degree of transparency and minimal animosity. Rather than taking an adversarial stance, which is common among many provider organizations, we have learned that when payers are approached as partners in treatment of their members, inevitable mistakes or missteps can be quickly rectified and ultimately the patient has a smoother treatment experience. We have found relationship building to be worth the investment in time and energy.

To serve as the "air-traffic" control for the Behavioral Health System of Care as a whole, keeping tabs on the availability of services and patient flow or movement through the system

The last role that our Admission Department undertakes is huge: that of "air-traffic" control for the Behavioral Health System of Care as a whole. In this role, it is their responsibility to keep tabs on the availability of all services in the system by monitoring patient flow and movement. Here, the Admissions Department functions like an airport's air-traffic controller, monitoring the take-offs and landings of multiple aircraft simultaneously. In like fashion, Admissions monitors who is coming into the system, who is going out as well as who is stepping up or stepping down from every level of care. It is a complicated task and even in a relatively small Behavioral Health System of Care, this job can be quite difficult, especially if the services are in high demand.

Behavioral health systems are highly dynamic environments and can change multiple times a day. Individual patient situations are subject to differing pressures and their symptoms and needs often change unpredictably. And as a system, there can be many competing needs from patients and families as well as from programs that change or go awry. It's not a matter of predictable logistics that unfold in a planful manner. Various constituencies, both internal to the system and external put pressure on the system for rapid change. In all instances, the challenge becomes the efficient management of patient transitions within the system while queuing up many who are waiting and eager for an admission. The art perhaps is doing all of this while maintaining the focus on customer service.

All this complexity is often most assisted with electronic databases that accept input from each program in the Behavioral Health System of Care. Designated individuals can update the databases in real time as events unfold, with built-in checks at set times throughout each day. Many organizations use electronic billboards or screens that show all the comings and goings, with open beds or slots clearly visible. These screens are extremely useful in the "command" center of the Admissions Department and can provide a ready visual in nursing offices or staff space at the programs. Input from the programs to the screens is used to communicate any discharge which in turn alerts the command center to the availability of space for a new admission.

Given how critical this function is to the system, we use a combination of additional methods to enhance communication. For instance, we begin every day with a "Flash" meeting which occurs at 8:30 every weekday in a Zoom room. The meeting includes leadership from all programs and is chaired by the Admissions Department. It is a quick meeting, usually lasting no more than fifteen minutes and includes a reporting of the actual census for each program (which is then verified by the program) along with any discharges planned for today or anticipated for the upcoming few days. Importantly, a member of the Utilization Review team is always present and provides updates on any potential payment risks due to insurance coverage for any patient in any program. This in turn alerts the program and the Admissions Department of any potential movement in the day ahead.

Another key part of the Admissions Department is a control function in which certain designated people are charged with the responsibility of approving admissions for each level of care. As there are often multiple patients waiting to admit or change from one level of care to another, these people need an accurate understanding of the clinical needs of each patient, and numerous issues related to internal and external advocacy, program capacity (including acuity), and business demands. All these concerns come into play in the decision-making and approval for any movement in the system. It should come as no surprise that the individuals who are charged with this responsibility have a very difficult task. They must balance reviewing and accepting patients who meet the clinical presentation that the System is designed to care for with the business reality of keeping the beds filled.

Example

Most systems struggle with lists of people they will not admit. Some of these are called "DNA lists," or even the fancier, "Persona Non Grata," but regardless of title, it is a slippery slope to make these decisions at the program level. As a long-practicing nurse once put it eloquently, "I have a unit of people to take care of here. Don't expect me to get excited about a new admission." A hospital had a large whiteboard in the staff lounge area. It was filled with names and next to each name was a date.

When a new administrator was hired with the mandate of increasing the census, the board was a logical place to start. "Who are all these people?" and "what are these dates?" The answer, somewhat sheepishly offered, was "these are the people that we will not readmit. And the dates are the day they left us never to return." Somewhat taken aback by the assured response, the new administrator pointed to one name near the center of the board. "Why can't that one return?" Someone else in the room shot back, "he was a discharge problem." The administrator pointed to another and again a quick response followed, "she was rude to a nurse, and we think stole things from other patients." The exercise went on with the message being clear: once you made the board, you weren't coming back. In fact, the board was so powerful that the process for an admission had evolved to include a review of the board. The new administrator removed the board.

Part of managing things like this is to designate a small group of individuals to manage admission decisions across the organization with the expectation that most requests for an admission are to be supported not denied. It's about getting to yes, even if qualifiers are needed. As a part of that, it is important to have a senior medical person, like the Chief Medical Officer, available to provide necessary medical oversight, but aside from that, admission is about getting people into programs not keeping them out. Over time, we have built a culture that truly believes that programs operate best when they are full and that everyone, even the "bad discharge problem" from a year ago deserves a second chance. People and situations do change and with that is the potential for readiness in treatment to shift. When we have a particular presentation for admission that may have ended poorly in a prior admission, we will convene a discussion with the potential admission and two members of the clinical staff to scope out the goals of this admission and to set some ground rules. It's usually a productive intervention and the result is an admission.

Treatment services in a Behavioral Health System of Care

Treatment services can be as varied and broad as there are diagnoses and alternative philosophies of treatment; in other words, the possibilities are nearly endless. The main point that we want to make in this section is that in a true Behavioral Health System of Care, the services are designed to fit the population being served and are linked one to another throughout the system to provide a rational pathway for recovery. Second, we strongly suggest that there are certain hallmarks of a good program or constellation of services. That is, regardless of treatment philosophy, we believe that there are strategies that can be used to improve the delivery of behavioral healthcare that are better than current practice.

We've spoken to the "Pillars" of a Behavioral Health System of Care, a main one being that treatment services are developed in such a way as to provide a rational road to recovery. In re-stating this core intent of a System in this section, we go into some further detail about related issues, including system focus, system design, and system continuity and similarly program focus, design, and continuity. Definitionally, we are using the term "system" to describe the "whole," which is the totality of services and programs under the administrative umbrella of a particular organization. The term "program" is used to describe the components or the "parts" of the larger system.

The issue of "focus" at both the system and program level is critical to the design and ultimate success of a Behavioral Health System of Care. Our observation is that most organizations calling themselves "systems" attempt to serve too broad an array of psychiatric and psychological conditions. A system can't be all things to all people and even when providing services of high quality, they often fail in their attempts to make a difference for a sizable portion of the population. This occurs because the population many are trying to treat is so diverse. When this occurs and programs attempt to respond to many types of needs, treatment becomes diffuse and ultimately unsuccessful. Psychiatric conditions, no different than general medical conditions, require treatment targeted for the issues and symptoms extant in the population. One of two things happen when the focus is poor: the system or program provides a generic form of treatment that has limited value to the patient, or the system or program provides a focused form of treatment that is successful with just a subset of the consumer population. In the latter instance, lack of success is often attributed to the "resistance" of the patient as opposed to the misdirection of the treatment.

So, what is an appropriate focus? The authors have been leaders in several organizations (systems of care) with different foci, including individuals with eating disorders, adolescents with severe family dysfunction, and adults with co-occurring severe mental illness and substance abuse. While each of these organizations targeted a broad population, they at least provided enough direction to build services, programs, and a system of care whose purpose is to understand the specific needs of that population and envision a path to recovery. The definition of focus can be population based, diagnosis based, or some combination, but the key point is that it does not include everyone with a behavioral health issue. In some ways, it's just as important to determine who the system is not the right place for so those individuals can find the care they need elsewhere.

There are some important benefits to arranging care in this way. The first is that over time, the people who provide the care, the clinicians, doctors, nurses, and others, get better at what they do because of experience but also because training can be more targeted to the issues and problems that arise during treatment. Secondly, the system itself can adapt as it discovers what patients need, developing new and different services that can fill any treatment gaps. Over time, the clinical pathway to recovery improves and new services are developed. Third, we have found a clinical advantage to having patients continuously exposed to others confronting similar problems as themselves. As many with a psychiatric illness suffer in private, a cohort in a treatment setting offers the opportunity to learn from each other as well as a decrease in the sense of isolation that often comes from living with a serious psychiatric condition.

Having established a population focus, we turn to design considerations, always keeping in mind that the raison d'etre, the reason for being, is to promote recovery from the disorders that we treat. The task is accomplished by developing a treatment road that utilizes clinical programs of varying intensity to assist individuals experiencing distress. This involves creating a well thought out path that progresses toward health, stability, and self-defined outcomes articulated by the patient and their family. We often think of this as "architecture," like a bridge or series of bridges that support the individual from one location to another to another until they get to their destination. The design process poses the development question of "what programs and services do individuals experiencing this type of psychiatric distress need to progress toward recovery?"

Earlier we discussed levels of care or treatment programs at varying levels of intensity that represent the components of a system. These often include inpatient or hospital care, residential care, sub-acute care such as partial hospital or day treatment and intensive outpatient treatment and outpatient care. Within each level of care, there can be multiple programs, many sub-types and even a range of services offered. In practice, systems of care tend to offer fewer options at the inpatient level and more options at the sub-acute and outpatient levels. Key determinants of this are the specific needs of the population and the availability of reimbursement.

While the treatment programs within any Behavioral Health System of Care can take many forms, the key ideas in design are:

1 Intentionality – the programs are designed to work together as a cohesive whole.
2 Constancy – the treatment philosophy, language, modalities of therapy, and general processes are similar across programs that constitute the system.
3 Continuity – the programs easily share information about the patient, the progress they've made, and their continuing needs as they move from one program to another. We call this the "hand-off" from one location to the next.

By designing clinical treatment according to these principles, we are taking responsibility as professionals and as a Behavioral Health System of Care overall, to make it as easy as possible for the patient and their family to understand and benefit from the services being provided. When services are not aligned, the patient carries the extra burden of trying to figure out what services they need, where to find and access them, and even how they should work. As a result, many patients lose any progress made in one program at the point of transition to another. By staying within a general set of treatment approaches and modalities, a well-conceived system reinforces skill and knowledge attainment from one level of care to the next. This allows the patient to build mastery of concepts, coping mechanisms, and life skills. A well-conceived Behavioral Health System of Care makes these transitions much smoother with the goal of being seamless.

Our point is that continuity or the repetition and reinforcement in a Behavioral Health System of Care is intentional and is enhanced in many ways, including a similar "look and feel" to all the system's programs. There are also specific tools and processes in place that have been designed to promote continuity. In most systems, a critical tool to continuity is an electronic health record (EHR). In this age, it goes without saying that programs within a Behavioral Health System of Care will utilize the same EHR, thereby allowing information from one level of care or program to easily be passed from one level of care to another. The attending clinicians in each level of care have access to records and communication from all prior treaters within the system.

While there is no doubt that this has enormous benefits in terms of information flow, it brings with it two important risks. One is simply the risk of an overabundance of information; clinicians have so much information at their fingertips that what they need to know is often hard to find. In such a sea of too much information, what is needed now can be hard to locate. Second, with the abundance of information available, there is a tendency for one program to assume the receiving program will know what they know (or at least have access to it). This can create a detachment between programs. The all-important "color" of a case, that which is often not written down, is lost.

At Walden, we also instituted a process called the "hand-off" to be used every time a patient moved from one level of care or program to another. The clinician from the sending program was responsible for reaching out and setting up an in-person, voice, or face-to-face (including Zoom, Teams, etc.) communication with the primary clinician in the receiving program. We feel strongly that voice mails, emails, and even EHR entries are not enough. *It was this live communication between two clinicians that provided the sharing of a level of detail and understanding about a patient that would otherwise have been missing that makes a difference.* Many times, impressions, things that worked to connect with the family and even things to avoid in trying to connect are not present or easily accessible in the EHR and are essential pieces for the receiving team. Additionally, we found that patients and their families found it reassuring to know that the treaters in both programs had conferred about them.

Program design in a system of care

The central question in program design is "what are you (the program) trying to accomplish?" It's a rather complicated question, though it is simplified to some degree within a Behavioral Health System of Care because the answer is really informed by decisions that have already been made. The overall focus of the system in terms of population served and the place or position that the program occupies within the system provide a clear sense of direction. If the program is a higher level of care (i.e. inpatient) issues of safety, symptom reduction, and readiness for treatment will often be primary. If the program is a lower level of care, issues related to specific therapeutic goals and the ability to sustain treatment progress after discharge will often be front and center. Each program within a Behavioral Health System of Care accrues its definition as the result of how it fits within that specific system and what the system overall expects it to accomplish. In essence, each program within a Behavioral Health System of Care defines its role and then owns a part of the recovery pathway Each program is a "steppingstone" or bridge to the next program.

Regardless of the particular focus of the program, we recommend several key practices within each program:

The use of interdisciplinary teams and team meetings

It's accepted in healthcare that treatment works best when there is good communication among all the professionals who are involved in the treatment of an individual. We talk a lot about how to improve this with most treatment settings using the popular term "multidisciplinary team" when describing the working and communication of the many providers involved in care. In behavioral health, these teams generally include groups of professionals representing different disciplines such as psychiatry, nursing, social work, and expressive therapy. The idea is that each member of the team contributes to the assessment and treatment of a patient so that communication flows easily so that collaborative treatment can begin.

In truth, while most health systems have some sort of team structure, they are often hierarchical, rigid, and operate with a top-down communication structure. Aligned with the medical model, membership in many systems is not equal and the input and authority of some greatly outweighs the contributions of others. We prefer the term "interdisciplinary team" and use it to indicate certainly that there are multiple professionals involved on the team but more importantly, that they are working in concert to develop an integrated plan for the patient. While a medical professional usually heads the team, we have had good success in creating a culture in which all members of the team have a voice and are heard. Everyone's contribution is valued.

For us, this is an issue of organizational culture and part of that culture is based on a commitment we make to recruit and hire individuals who want to work in a team-oriented setting. In interviews, we ask questions about personal experience with teams, and specifically about a professional's ability to work alongside other professionals as a team member. Such questioning informs us about the candidate but also communicates to the potential member the essence of the job and the culture we are looking to maintain. If we are talking to someone who does better working autonomously, both parties can discern quickly that this might not be the best setting for them.

We also ask if an individual is "curious." It's a great interview question because again it speaks directly to our culture. It often leads to a discussion about the illnesses we treat and the reality that while no one has solved the puzzle yet, we are collaboratively working on it. Ultimately, the question becomes an invitation to become curious with us, to join our work, and most importantly that all contributions will be welcomed.

Some components of treatment must involve the family (family therapy, counseling, psychoeducation) or others in the person's natural environment

Treatment and life itself do not take place in a vacuum. When an individual has taken steps to make life changes by seeking care, it's important to assess how these changes will be supported by and ultimately impact their social world. For individuals struggling with a complex behavioral health illness, it is often the individuals in their social system, specifically, parents, spouses or partners, friends, co-workers, etc. who make the difference in moving toward recovery. Supportive family and social connections are essential to recovery. In fact, we tell our patients that no one can recover on their own. It must be a team effort. The challenge, however, for many of the people we work with is that due to the longevity and severity of their illness, many natural supports have fallen away. Even if some are still involved as a family or social support resource, they are often so frustrated with the failings of the mental health system that calls from a treating clinician go unanswered. Time in a program becomes time away and not a true opportunity for change.

A first step in any case is to identify and engage any support that the patient identifies. Many programs send out invitations to family meetings or family therapy, especially if the patient is young and living at home; but we recommend these meetings for people of all ages. In our experience, when loved ones or supports are identified, they often tell us that they have been left in the dark in past treatments. They have no idea how to help the individual make the needed behavior adjustments for the life changes they seek. We work to engage the support system in a range of services, from intensive family therapy with a focus on issues in a single family to family psychoeducation which focuses on general understanding of specific conditions, medications, and complications. When families and other significant people are included in the treatment and discharge planning, there is a much greater likelihood of successful transition to home.

A full schedule of group and other therapies that promote recovery, reinforce treatment-related goals and objectives, and create a momentum toward sustainable functioning post-discharge

We are firm believers in providing a full, active curriculum of groups and therapeutic events throughout the treatment day, including weekends Strong clinical programs publish their schedules weekly, update them often, and engage professionals of all types in carrying out an assortment of group therapies. The components of the treatment schedule will be based upon the problems and issues that the program is intended to address, though we have found it useful to create a balance of skills-based learning groups, process (talking) groups, and expressive therapy groups. We recommend a heavy core emphasis on education about the diagnoses being treated, coping skills development, and additional "electives" which patients choose (with input from the treatment team) from a menu of relevant activities. Group therapies should teach elements of evidence-based practices (i.e. cognitive behavior therapy) extrapolated from known evidence-based practices and widely accepted core treatment philosophies or approaches (i.e. 12-step model). These groups are offered multiple times per week with topics that vary over the course of treatment depending on the average length of stay for patients utilizing the program.

We have had remarkable success with the addition of an Expressive Therapies program which is targeted to assisting individuals in nonverbal mediums. These select groups focus on maintaining health and balance in life and include yoga, mindfulness, art therapy, and dance movement. For many individuals struggling with long-term illnesses, expressive therapies offer a very different approach from conventional "talking" treatment and are restorative. We have seen remarkable results.

A pre-discharge meeting with the patient to review the course of treatment and to establish recommendations for follow-up or next steps and ultimately to develop a plan for discharge

Historically, discharging from a behavioral health program has been a lot like jumping off a cliff. You are never sure how or where you're going to land. Recognizing discharge as a critical moment in the treatment process, it is unfortunate that it is often poorly managed especially in programs with short lengths of stay. While many patients are eager for discharge especially when they are moving out of an inpatient or residential setting, there are several important activities that should take place to ensure that the patient is truly ready, that there is a good plan in place that the patient agrees with which defines next steps in treatment, and that the transition to that next step has every chance of succeeding.

It is almost always best when the treatment team and the patient have advanced knowledge of discharge and agree as to the patient's readiness and the aftercare plan. In a well-conceived Behavioral Health System of Care, many patients will be stepping down to another program in the same system and therefore have the advantage of receiving some advanced orientation to the new setting. We create opportunities for the patient and family to ask questions about the program, see where they are going, and ideally to meet briefly with the new clinician assigned to work with them. This prep work is particularly helpful for individuals and families who are anxious about the next step in care. Any opportunity to anticipate concerns and make a human connection to the new setting prior to the formal discharge can make all the difference.

From the organization's standpoint, this works best when both the sending and receiving clinician have a working knowledge of the receiving program and ideally the staff that work in it. We have always encouraged our clinical staff to visit and even work for periods of time in different levels of care. It is invaluable in creating an awareness of the program nuances and allows for an accurate and personal endorsement. The more program staff know clinicians in other programs, the more they can convey the warmth and connection that patients' need as they step into a transition in care.

References

Aarons, G. A., Hurlburt, M., and Horwitz, S. M. (2011). Advancing a conceptual model of evidence-based practice implementation in public service sectors. *Administration and Policy in Mental Health and Mental Health Services Research*, 38(1), 4–23.

Davidson, L., O'Connell, M., Tondora, J., Lawless, M., and Evans, A. C. (2005). Recovery in serious mental illness: A new wine or just a new bottle? *Professional Psychology: Research and Practice*, 36(5), 480–487.

Drake, R. E., Merrens, M. R., and Lynde, D. W. (2005). *Evidence-Based Mental Health Practice: A Textbook.* W.W. Norton & Company.

Mee-Lee, D., Shulman, G. D., Fishman, M., Gastfriend, D. R., and Griffith, J. H. (eds.) (2001). *ASAM PPC-2R: ASAM Patient Placement Criteria for the Treatment of Substance-Related Disorders*, Second Edition Revised. American Society of Addiction Medicine.

Schein, E. H. (2010). *Organizational Culture and Leadership*, 4th Edition. Jossey-Bass.

Substance Abuse and Mental Health Services Administration (SAMHSA). (2016). SAMHSA's Working Definition of Recovery: 10 Guiding Principles of Recovery. Substance Abuse and Mental Health Services Administration.

Torrey, W. C., Drake, R. E., Dixon, L., Burns, B. J., Flynn, L., Rush, A. J., Clark, R. E., and Klatzker, D. (2001). Implementing evidence-based practices for persons with severe mental illnesses. *Psychiatric Services*, 52(1), 45–50.

6

RULES OF THE ROAD

Key Operating Principles in a Behavioral Health System of Care

Patient care within healthcare systems is a multifaceted endeavor, characterized by intricate interactions among healthcare professionals, patients, families, and the broader healthcare infrastructure. Effective patient care necessitates seamless collaboration and communication among diverse healthcare professionals, including physicians, nurses, pharmacists, and allied health professionals (Wei et al. 2020). Research indicates that interdisciplinary teamwork enhances patient safety, quality of care, and clinical outcomes (Manser 2009). However, achieving optimal collaboration requires addressing hierarchical barriers, fostering mutual respect, and promoting open communication channels.

Transitions between care settings, such as hospitals, primary care, and home care, pose significant challenges to patient safety and care coordination. Poorly managed transitions contribute to medication errors, duplicative testing, and gaps in follow-up care (Coleman 2003). Implementing standardized protocols or rules can mitigate risks associated with care transitions, ensuring seamless continuity of care and reducing adverse events.

Addressing the complexities of patient care requires a holistic approach that prioritizes collaboration, innovation, and continuous quality improvement. By embracing patient-centered principles and leveraging technological advancements, healthcare organizations can optimize care delivery, enhance patient experiences, and improve health outcomes.

Perhaps more than most healthcare systems, Behavioral Health Systems of Care have an extra degree of complexity. They're constructed to provide an array of services to individuals with serious psychiatric conditions and employ

DOI: 10.4324/9781315177366-7

many (hopefully) talented and committed individuals to deliver these services. Even under the best of conditions and with excellent staffing, there may be a variety of possible treatment approaches. Added to that are the strong opinions of behavioral health providers each espousing their own model of care. This becomes increasingly so with complicated cases.

To manage this complexity and to provide a sense of internal consistency relative to both operations and mission, it is incumbent on each Behavioral Health System of Care to establish some standard operating principles or "rules of the road." These rules can serve as an operating standard for all care in the system but become essential when there are higher level needs or challenges in a case. The "rules" discussed in this chapter reflect our thinking based on our own experience and experimentation over forty years through three different organizations serving three distinctly different clinical populations. And while our short list is not an exhaustive one, each of the rules we identify may need to be altered or adapted for a variety of reasons. Regardless, we do believe that having clear rules that are known and practiced throughout the organization is essential. We recommend these as a starting point at least.

Rule #1: There is one admission for the entire episode of care

One of the most important advantages of a system of care for patients and families is that once admitted – to any level of care – the patient has access to all the resources and programs that exist in the system. They can move within the system to different levels of care without having to "re-apply" for admission; there is no additional entering and exiting. This is important as in a treatment episode many patients and families will utilize multiple programs and levels of care as their care unfolds. Access to the system's resources and programs must be easy and streamlined in order to manage any of these transitions.

In practice, transitions in care occur whether the treatment progresses smoothly or not. We have found that not infrequently, progress toward health and well-being does not follow a predicted path and it is never linear. This means that for many patients progressing from one level of care to a lower level of care is not like walking down a staircase. As a patient's needs change, with some setbacks and anticipated difficulty, the patient may require a "step up" to a higher intensity program, sometimes even one that they have already progressed through previously. When this situation occurs, *it is the responsibility of the current treatment team to facilitate the transition with the patient and family by determining what is the appropriate next step in the episode of care and to facilitate a seamless transition to that program or level of care to best fit the needs of the patient at that time.*

While this may seem like the obvious thing to do, it is, in fact, not what generally happens when people seek services. In most healthcare systems, when a patient is having trouble in a level of care, they and their family must fend for themselves. The patient may even be unceremoniously discharged and left on their own to find a new program or additional resources to move forward. When a patient no longer fits the program in which they were being treated, the message of treatment failure can permeate the experience. Sometimes, with a referral or suggestions, patients are required to search for a new program on their own and then apply for admission. This creates chaos and insecurity for the patient and the family.

In a Behavioral Health System of Care, we follow the rule that transitions within the system, including transitions where the patient takes a "step back," are an expected part of the treatment experience and must be easily facilitated. They are normalized and explained as needed time-limited interventions to support a patient through a challenging time, never as a failure in treatment. There is no requirement to find a new program nor to re-apply as all movement between levels of care is facilitated by the holding treatment team and managed internally by the system. A transition should not be a burden to the patient or family.

Example

Karen R had a long history of mental health treatments and entered our system in an acute psychiatric crisis. She was admitted to our inpatient unit due to escalated eating disorder behaviors and several recent incidents of self-harm. In the past, these events quickly became more serious and were often severe enough to be life threatening. As a result, her presentation made her challenging for other systems to hold. In truth, she and her family had come to believe that no system could really treat her, most would merely hold her for a while and then discharge her home until things escalated again.

Her work on our inpatient unit was slow but productive. She was able to restore weight, and working with her clinician came to understand that there was a relationship between gaining weight and her feeling self-destructive. She learned to recognize when she was having self-destructive thoughts, and most importantly, she was able to identify when she would get to the point of feeling the need to act on them. After a period of relative stability, her inpatient treatment team, working with her family, agreed that a step down to the system's residential program made sense.

Recognizing the need to anticipate and creatively plan for her self-destructive acts was a concern for the residential program, the sending team on the inpatient unit, and her family. From the perspective of the residential program, they needed assurance from Karen that she could work with them when she was getting to the point where she felt the need to act on a self-destructive thought and would be willing to let them help. And with the inpatient team, there was a need for a plan that could be implemented quickly so that if Karen reported an intense need to be self-destructive, they could move in quickly and help her manage her safety. And from the family, unfortunately came the belief based on their past experiences that any transition in care was really a discharge out of the program. Such scenarios were all too familiar as they were convinced that the system was getting ready to discharge her outright and wash their hands of her case.

As with many complex cases, before anything was put into play, the inpatient team convened a meeting which included the residential program leadership and the family. Rather than taking the stand that Karen would not feel the need to self-harm, they anticipated that those strong feelings would of course return. They anticipated that Karen would experience a desire to return to old and familiar behaviors as she continued to progress in recovery from her eating disorder. The challenge to the group was to work together to safely manage those strong feelings and to work with Karen to decrease them over time.

What resulted was a commitment from Karen to speak directly to her residential team when she felt the need to act on a self-destructive thought. The residential team agreed to first try to manage the experience in the program with extra clinical time, but if that didn't work to rapidly facilitate a step up back to the inpatient unit. And the inpatient unit agreed to facilitate the rapid step up, even if that meant going over census, and then to maintain Karen on the inpatient unit just long enough to allow her to stabilize and then to transfer her back to the residential program. The clinical framework was reviewed and understood by all: that a step up was not a treatment failure but rather a success in managing strong feelings by giving Karen the support she needs. Her family, never having felt held through these events in the past, was speechless.

Importantly, Karen's insurance provider was also on board with the plan. Over time, they had developed a working trust of the system and knew that any step up to the inpatient unit, although costly, was clearly needed and would be time limited. They trusted that all parties were working to move Karen forward into less restrictive treatments and agreed to authorize whatever level of care the team felt they needed to maintain Karen's safety.

Rule #2: Patients who are currently being treated in the system receive priority for program access over patients outside of the system

As a Behavioral Health System of Care grows, it will inevitably encounter times when the service system is in such high demand that it can impede patients entering and exiting the system. This disrupts the "flow of the system" and creates periods of "grid lock," meaning that the overall volume in one or more components of the system is so high that it impedes movement of patients through other levels of care. Two significant problems result, both related to access. The first is that patients currently in the system cannot easily move to the next level of care and their progress is slowed as bottlenecks occur. We found this to occur most often in acute levels of care where patients having trouble in a lower level of care cannot be easily and quickly "stepped up." The second problem relates to new patients, those who have never been in the system before, who experience enormous difficulty gaining entry to the system. They wait, often at home with family members or in other programs that struggle to hold them in an untenable situation.

We experienced this firsthand at Walden Behavioral Care during the Covid pandemic between 2020 and 2022. With a sudden increase in the need for acute services and programming, leaders in the Admissions Department and managers in various programs did their best to balance the needs of all parties and to try to accommodate requests for admission at a time when the constriction in staffing impacted the number of discharges that occurred. The Admissions Department developed and juggled waitlists and worked diligently to anticipate any upcoming discharges and to prioritize needs for the limited openings that were in programs. Despite all their efforts, nothing seemed to stem the high demand or relieve the paralysis that existed from within the system. Families and outside providers became impatient. Not only was our Admissions Team attempting a difficult juggling act, but many of our staff began to experience the ethical dilemma of weighing the needs of one patient and family against the needs of another. It was not a comfortable place to be.

After a while, it became clear that waiting for the situation to "level out" or return to normal was not a solution. With a group of senior leaders, we established a plan that was used to guide the order of priorities in making any movement decision. We chose to favor current patients, those in our system, and prioritized their movement into other levels of care over patients not yet in the system and waiting for admission. It was our hope that the delay for those outside of the system would be only a matter of days, but we found that especially during periods of high demand, the wait could be weeks long, sometimes even months.

At one point, when the situation became particularly acute, we added the step of a two to one ratio plan to guide admissions. This meant that for every two internal patients moved within the system, one external patient was admitted. This important strategy was critical as it allowed some new patients to enter the system while affording our leadership time to address the slow movement from within. Of course, as with any rule, this was not absolute. The chief clinical and program officers, the CMO and COO, were able to override any decision based on their judgment of patient need and their assessment of what the system could tolerate. While not perfect, it did provide a general rule and system expectation that supported the organization's mission and values to fully treat patients in the system as our number one priority. And at the same time, by continuing to facilitate entry to the system, albeit on a reduced basis, we recognized and addressed the need for new patients to be able to access the care that they require.

Rule #3: Once a patient, always a patient

This "rule," sometimes stated as the mantra "*we never give up*," speaks to a key value of the organization to practice resilience and "hold hope" for any patient that we treat. We acknowledge that recovery is rarely a linear experience and for some can be a long and difficult road. Over the course of the illness, many may need to return to the system for additional support and treatment numerous times. It is the opposite attitude of a practice that we have seen in other places where the organization or program keeps an active "DNA" or "DO NOT ADMIT" list for patients who have been determined to be too difficult or troublesome.

A key distinction is that rather than see the need for additional treatment as "failure," of the last treatment or the patient, the Behavioral Health System of Care recognizes the longer "journey" that some individuals require as well as the capacity for people to change over time. Because of this, we accept responsibility for providing treatment that is individualized and effective each time a patient is presented with a desire for additional care. This may challenge the system to reconceptualize its approach from thinking of each admission as a discrete event to the longer orientation of episodic treatment. We do this hopefully in coordination with what the patient and family have experienced and are motivated to pursue, but for us internally, it requires our staff to welcome back past patients in a non-blaming way and to work to engage a returning patient in taking the next step forward rather than seeing a re-admission as a failure.

In accepting this responsibility, the treatment team and program must avoid the tendency to "blame" the patient for having the disease or disorder that they are struggling with and must understand their own feelings of frustration. It is essential that all treaters orient instead to the need to support the positive personal attributes of the patient to progress and recover and most importantly their willingness to continue in their struggle. Embracing these values as an organization has widespread impact on individual staff as they are clearly expected to maintain a positive attitude as they work with patients and to provide support for them if they begin to waver in their hope for the patient's recovery.

Example

We were fortunate to have a visit from a former patient who after years of struggling with her illness had recovered. Her story was quite miraculous, having been in treatment for over a decade. Since her recovery, she had begun speaking publicly about her experience in treatment to raise awareness. As a part of that effort, she agreed to speak with our clinical staff about her struggle with her illness and the very personal experience of treatment over so much time. Our clinicians listened intently as she remembered her adolescent years and how the illness developed, led to an acute admission, and then to a series of readmissions over many years.

She spoke about the power of the treatment relationships she had formed with providers and how their support was a primary force in her recovery. She recalled coming to a point where she felt her own resolve to persevere and not give up during some dark days. She acknowledged that there were some very trying times for her and her family. It was clear that she appreciated the commitment that the system had made to her and told the group that she never felt that she was totally on her own. She came to realize that she could come back when she needed to, and, most importantly, didn't feel negatively judged for not being a quick recovery.

As she neared the end of her presentation, she asked if there were any questions. There was a moment of respectful silence and then one clinician leaned forward and asked,

> You said you were hospitalized ten times. That seems like a lot. Which hospitalization was the most helpful, the one that made the difference?

Without missing a beat, our speaker responded, "the first."

She went on to explain that it was the first time walking through the doors that was the hardest for her. That was the first time she had to acknowledge to herself that things were out of control and that she needed someone to help her. She knew she couldn't do it on her own. And it was in that first admission that she felt that commitment that the system offered her and her family. She said that it helped to hear that they would not need to be alone in their struggle moving forward.

Rule #4: A patient's current treatment team decides the next step in treatment

We really regard this as the "golden rule" in the Behavioral Health System of Care as it creates a clear locus for decision-making and an expectation about the next step in treatment which ultimately relieves much of the anxiety that is associated in an organization with any discussion about discharge. In fact, absent this rule, most treatment teams spend way too much time on the critical questions of "where will this person go next," and most importantly, "who gets to make that decision." From the perspective of other programs in the system, this attention is often directed toward protecting their own gates that lead to an admission. Left undecided and ambiguous, programs spend an enormous amount of time trying to anticipate who might present for an admission and assessing whether the patient is a "good fit" for the program. While this form of self-protection is understandable, it does not serve the system well. Clarifying who makes the decision about the next step in treatment cuts through all of that and is often common sense. Our rule is that the treatment team that is currently treating the patient is responsible for determining where in the system the patient will move to next.

In fairness, most of the time these treatment decisions aren't a big problem. They are routinely made at the program level by the assigned treatment team with little or no fanfare. Movement in the system is often anticipated and the flow of the system, patients stepping up and stepping down, works well with patients ending up in the correct level of care. However, there are times when a particularly challenging patient or a difficult program situation presents itself. It is at these times that it becomes evident that there can be tremendous pushback, even in a well-run system. When it occurs, it almost always has to do with a situation in which there is a specific behavior or cluster of behaviors and the perception of a heightened level of risk that is uncomfortable for the receiving program. Often, there is a sense of fear.

This is not unlike what happens between larger health systems and unrelated programs that are always wary of what is known in the industry as a "dump." These are referrals or transfers of a patient that is complex, perhaps aggressive, and almost always hard to fit into a specific program. They can be perceived as non-compliant or disinterested in treatment and often come with a risk for injury to self or others. To avoid the mistake of admitting one of these complex patients, many programs tend to adopt operational procedures that are self-protective. Sometimes, these are secretly folded into their admissions evaluation process, and at other times, can be much more transparent and known throughout the organization.

In a Behavioral Health System of Care, there is no admissions process through which a referral or step down can be stopped, but there is a transition process where important clinical information is exchanged. This is the point when the decision-making of the referring team may be questioned. Frequently, these situations involve patients stepping down from hospital level care and moving into some form of community-based treatment. The question at hand is always some version of "is this patient truly ready and/or safe enough to step down to a less restrictive program?"

Of course, it can also occur in the other direction, with a patient stepping up from a lower level of care back to the hospital. In this instance, the message is often, "we can't handle this patient and provide for their needs in a community-based program; we've done everything we can at this point." Often attached to the message is the spoken or subtle messaging that once the patient is out of the program, the patient is not welcome back. The door is closed.

When these situations do occur, we regard it as a clinical crisis that must be resolved in the best interests of the patient. It is important that the organization's leaders support the general rule that gives the decision-making to the "holding" program and treatment team. It must be assumed that these are the clinicians that are most knowledgeable and current with the condition of the patient *at this moment*. However, in a Behavioral Health System of Care, there is an opportunity for all involved in the case to come together for an honest and direct review of the case and the impediments that are being experienced in the transition. What is different however is that no program has the option of saying "no, we will not treat the patient." In the classic terminology of Dialectical Behavioral Therapy, the discussion is focused not on "no," rather "yes, and how ..."

This is likely accomplished with the Chief Clinical Officer or Chief Medical Officer's involvement. He or she meets with both sides of the transfer discussion to understand the patient's needs, including the presenting limiting problem, and understands the challenge this case presents to the program. Ultimately, the goal is to facilitate a clinically creative process in which both teams work together to find the best solution. The consultation provided reviews the critical issues with an understanding that all views have some truth and to the reality that there is no perfect solution. What is often the case with this type of closer scrutiny, or second opinion, is a change in stance, one that is more in line with a "yes, but" statement. This means that the obstacles to movement must be removed with some form of clinical accommodation or infusion of additional resources for a resolution to develop. Often, this process results in the receiving team feeling heard and supported with additional resources that make it more possible to meet the patient's needs.

Example

GW was an individual known throughout the substance use system who had struggled for years with a serious addiction problem and intermittent suicidal behavior. He was a frequent admission to the acute care hospital where he would inevitably end up after a serious suicide attempt. When not in the hospital, he settled, for a time, in our community-based Partial Hospital program. When he was doing well, the Partial Hospital Program seemed to be able to hold him, although the unpredictability of his personal safety made the staff nervous. They often said they felt as though they were holding a ticking time bomb.

Seemingly out of the blue, GW made a serious suicide attempt one afternoon after he had left the Partial Hospital Program. He was rushed to the emergency department in the local hospital where doctors and nurses revived him. He narrowly escaped death and after spending a week on a medical unit, he was transferred into our acute behavioral health facility. Almost as soon as he was admitted, the hospital got an unceremonious email from the Partial Hospital Program saying that they had come to the decision that GW should not return to their program. Although they said it with some clinical rationale, in essence they were bowing out.

In follow-up conversations, they talked about the emotional toll that the recent attempt had taken on their staff. They had a growing concern that they simply could not keep him safe.

Uncharacteristic of how transitions in care are usually handled in the system and feeling a strong discharge block, the inpatient team asked for a consultation with the Chief Clinical Officer and the Chief Medical Officer. Both interviewed GW and reviewed his chart. A meeting was convened with the inpatient team and the outpatient staff at the Partial Program.

These are important meetings even though they rarely result in finding a perfect solution. They are based on the system's rule that the holding team makes the disposition plan, and as a part of that, no program in the system can refuse to participate and opt out of a transfer. The meetings allow for all sides to voice their concerns with the effort to re-craft the problem as a system challenge rather than the burden of one program in the system. Part of the discussion is focused on asking each program to think creatively about a solution.

The Partial Hospital Program spoke to the unpredictability of GW's behavior and their very real fear that he would eventually die under their watch. They used a common logic in behavioral health, designating his behavior as a "psychiatric problem" and not a substance use problem. As a part of a substance use system, they said he was a bad fit for their program. Most importantly, they talked about their fear that he was simply too risky to be maintained in a community-based program. And the inpatient unit, while sympathetic to the Partial Program, did not see keeping GW in a locked hospital as a viable, long-term solution. And they countered that diagnostic presentations are often co-occurring disorders and saw little value in creating an exclusion based on GW's behavior.

After much discussion, the Chief Medical Officer summarized the problem and engaged the group in thinking creatively about what would be needed to add a layer of safety for GW. Together, each program compromised. A discharge plan developed that would have GW move into a sober living home for additional support and structure. With that in place, the Partial Hospitalization Program felt more comfortable working with GW and agreed to meet privately every day with GW daily to monitor his current level of suicidal thinking. And the inpatient unit made the commitment that if GW were to be determined to be at high risk for self-harm, he would be prioritized for the next inpatient bed.

Rule #5: Transitions between programs are always complicated and require verbal communication between the sending clinician and the receiving clinician

We place a premium on person-to-person communication particularly during the challenging time of a transition in level of care. The opportunity to create a personal communication between the patient's sending clinician to the receiving clinician is invaluable and almost always decreases the anxiety of the patient and their family. Most of the patients and families we've worked with will talk openly about the many obstacles they face moving from a program they have grown to know and likely trusted to one they have never heard of with people they don't know. It helps tremendously if they can see and feel the relationships they have formed being passed from a known person to a warm connection in the next level of care. We find that this person-to-person communication is essential despite the plethora of information available in electronic health records these days. In short, absent a verbal discussion between clinicians, most receiving clinicians and programs will base their understanding of a patient on a sanitized synopsis that they read in a medical record or heard secondhand. In both instances, much of the tone and "color" of a case is missed, particularly the ability for a sending clinician to present their client in a realistic and hopeful manner.

Of course, this direct communication is hard to do. All clinicians are busy, and we often hear how difficult it is to align schedules for a meaningful discussion. Added to that are the mechanics of connecting given the many modes of communication available today. Having a verbal discussion requires a commitment on the part of both parties and persistence. We've landed on a process that helps. It requires the sending clinician to email to the receiving program, usually to the attention of the clinical director. It is then the responsibility of the Clinical Director to get the information to the newly assigned clinician at the receiving program. In that email, the sending clinician briefly provides four things.

1 Their name and their best contact phone number along with some preferred times
2 A one sentence update on the presenting problem
3 A brief update on any safety concerns
4 Any thoughts about how to best help the patient to manage their anxiety at this transition (what has worked in the past)

Though time-consuming, it has been clear that the effort made by both sides of this transfer is worth it. Families feel held and liken the effort to "going the extra" mile to ensure that the transition works. And the patient appreciates the effort to pass along the relationship to the next group involved in their treatment. It creates buy-in at a time when many episodes of care fall apart.

Rule #6: We operate with a willingness to flex or adapt our services to meet the needs of the patient and their family

Healthcare systems are rigid, and large systems of care tend to be very rigid. At the core of that rigidity is a long-held belief that health providers know what is best for their patients, and more subtly, that patients should do as they are told. But this is changing, particularly with the increase in healthcare information now easily accessed by the public. Individuals and families know more about their symptoms and illnesses and as a result are less willing to do what they are told. Many present to a healthcare system having researched their problem and with an already formed idea of what they want, including how much of it and when. Added to that, individuals who present with more complex challenges often come with at least one experience, sometimes more, of how healthcare has failed them. They are skeptical and sometimes angry about what has not worked in the past and as a result are sensitive to moving forward with customary and usual treatment options.

As a Behavioral Health System of Care, we've learned that it is important to be flexible. Disagreement is not a bad thing and, in many cases, has turned into the beginning of a productive treatment relationship. As a system of care, we can easily accommodate opinions that may differ from ours and have found in many ways that it makes good clinical and business sense. When we assess a patient and make a recommendation for a level of care, we see that simply as our recommendation. We could be wrong, and patients often challenge our assessment and recommendation and then seek to modify what we've recommended to meet their own needs and the needs of their family. Because we have many levels of care and an ease of movement between them, we are often willing to try a level of care that might not make sense to us initially. If things go well, that's all for the good. It is after all, what we all want. And if things falter and the need for a higher level of care becomes evident, we can make that change quickly, often with the patient's agreement.

Example

Susan J presented to our intake department with her mother. After the interview, both met with the evaluator and who reviewed the key data points of her struggle with an eating disorder and made the recommendation for inpatient level of care. Susan and her mother reacted with surprise and almost immediately pushed back. Susan had commitments in her life and had tried inpatient treatment in the past and not only found it of little value. She said it felt like jail to her and had no intention of admitting. The evaluator calmly asked if Susan would be willing to problem solve a bit, and with her agreement, went back over the data of her evaluation, including her expected body weight, the behaviors she was engaging in and their frequency and asked Susan what her plan would be to address these if not in a hospital along with the genuine query of how the system could best support her.

Susan and her mother were taken aback. They had anticipated an argument, not problem solving, and the conversation turned into an honest dialog of what

Susan felt she could handle on her own and what she could readily identify what she needed help with. Ultimately, all agreed that Susan would try to manage some of her behaviors on her own and would attend a virtual partial hospital program for support in the work needed to increase her level of nutrition. She agreed to weekly monitoring by her Primary Care Clinician, and most importantly, to reconsider a brief hospitalization if the plan was not working. At the end of the discussion and planning, Susan commented that she thought she was coming in for an evaluation and instead felt as though she had embarked on a new treatment episode in which she was driving her care. She and her mother departed informed of the current state of her illness. For Susan, treatment was off to a good start; she felt heard throughout the evaluation and engaged in the system.

References

Coleman, E. A. (2003). Improving the quality of transitional care for persons with complex care needs. *Journal of the American Geriatrics Society*, 51(4), 449–555.

Manser, T. (2009). Teamwork and patient safety in dynamic domains of healthcare: A review of the literature. *Acta Anaesthesiologica Scandinavica*, 53(2), 143–151.

Wei, H., Corbett, R. W., Ray, J., and Wei, T. L. (2020). A culture of caring: The essence of healthcare interprofessional collaboration. *Journal of Interprofessional Care*, 34(3), 324–331.

7

CULTURE

The People Make It Work

Making a Behavioral Health System of Care work as it should is not just about hiring good people which, of course, is always necessary for any successful endeavor. It's about how to maximize an individual's inherent motivation to do this hard and rewarding work and to do it in a way that furthers the momentum of a well-conceived Behavioral Health System of Care. This is not a new concept; Deci and Ryan (1985) and others have discussed the many intrinsic factors that contribute to motivation. It's about developing what we call "the core," that group of individuals who make the organization their professional home and provide stability over time. As we consider this, we pay close attention to the ways in which we encourage their involvement in the continuous shaping of the organization so that they develop what we call "ownership." These are really strategies designed to support employees' continued growth as people and as behavioral health clinicians. We encourage collegial contact that creates a culture of support which we call the "social glue" of the organization and the way that leadership communicates appreciation and value for every job category and employee.

Wherever people congregate in a continuous manner, social systems form. The importance of social systems in shaping individual behavior has long been recognized (Parsons 1951). In a brief period, these social systems develop a series of rules, norms, and distinct subgroups (Schein 2010) and even assign roles to the individuals that are part of it. It makes sense that organizations, institutions, and companies form workplace environments which are, indeed, their own social systems. Each comes with some rules and norms prescribed by the owners and leaders.

DOI: 10.4324/9781315177366-8

The people in these organizations, usually the employees, react to the conditions in which they live and work and form subgroups, each with their own ways of behaving. Part of that is to accomplish the assigned tasks of the organization or workplace, but they also form opinions, attitudes, and beliefs about all aspects of their daily working lives. It's this unseen, intangible web of human responses that can be said to be the "culture" of the workplace and it is very powerful.

Our view is that "culture" and the nurturing of specific attributes of culture are critical in environments where healthcare is provided, and that this is especially true in behavioral health. The behavioral healthcare environment is largely defined by the "culture of healing" (or a lack of a culture of healing) and is the place where people in significant emotional distress try to get better. Each person being treated is seeking a pathway to healing which always involves some sort of difficult change that they are asked to make.

In addition, people seeking behavioral health services almost always arrive in a heightened emotional state and often under duress. Many experience an added pressure of an implied expectation to be "quiet about it" due to the associated stigma involved. This can be compounded when an individual experiences a lack of sensitivity to their racial, ethnic, religious or gender identity, or sexual orientation. It is always incumbent on the organization to foster a sense of awareness and sensitivity among all providers.

We know that recovery from a moderate to severe behavioral health disorder is often more complicated and less formulaic than other forms of medical treatment and recovery. In most instances, the patient who may be entering treatment at the insistence of another must not only agree to the treatment but "engage" in the treatment for change to occur. In behavioral health, treatment is not just "done to you" as in having a surgery or setting a broken bone but done *with you as an active participant*. This requires *motivation* and motivation requires some sense of being able to achieve a positive outcome.

Sometimes, we call this "hope," and we know that having a sense of hope is often the beginning of recovery. Most people in treatment are aided in approaching complex, difficult tasks by having another person supporting them in the effort and giving them the sense that there is hope. "This time things will be different." For providers, the individuals involved in the delivery of behavioral healthcare services and who carry out many complex tasks of treatment, it is the way these tasks are done and what is communicated between the staff and patients in the process that is most impacted by culture. The famous quote often attributed to the poet, Maya Angelou has resonance here: "I've learned that people will forget what you said, people will forget what you did, but people will never forget how you made them feel."

Properties of culture

We have found that the culture of a behavioral health organization has a profound impact on staff and patients alike. But culture does not just happen. It is methodically built over time by the concerted effort of leadership. It is the relationship between leadership and staff and between various subgroups of staff with each other that creates the dominant characteristics of a particular work environment and its culture. The impact on patients is really a by-product of what is happening and affecting the people who work in these environments. Once formed, most work cultures are static for extended periods of time. But they can change quickly and intermittently as they are acutely responsive to major changes impacting the organization. The changes can include a new CEO, a sudden change in economic conditions (both to the good and bad), extreme workplace events (i.e. a patient death), and major alterations of the work environment like workforce shortages and other strong external factors (i.e. the Covid pandemic).

Despite the tendency of some to consider culture more of an afterthought, there is really no area of work life that is not impacted in some way by the culture of the organization and there are often sub-cultures that arise in specific subgroups. Leadership and management are always a major source of cultural norms, and this occurs whether they "believe" or not in the existence of culture. For instance, if a leadership group is unconcerned about the organization's culture, the result can be as impactful and perhaps even more so, than a leadership group that recognizes and works to shape an organizational culture. The decision to ignore culture, either actively or benignly, is an important determinant of employee behavior and work satisfaction. In behavioral health, such a decision almost always works out badly and becomes a limiting factor in the success of the organization.

Most social systems, including work environments and subgroups, can be quite powerful. Subgroups form around some kernel of common identity; it could be a work location, a shared job function, a professional designation, or seniority or tenure. Each subgroup allows its members to enjoy a sense of belonging and sometimes a sense of "specialness" because of their shared identity. The bonding of members in a subgroup is a natural and expected occurrence in almost any organization and is presumed to be healthy for the organization if coalescing doesn't become an obstacle for participating positively in the dominant culture of the organization or puts one subgroup at odds with another in a detrimental competitive relationship.

In behavioral healthcare, it's particularly important for management to have a good understanding of who comprises the workforce and most importantly why they chose to work in this field as a basis for shaping culture. It is a question we routinely ask in staff meetings to foster a sense of common purpose. It is also critically important to understand what subgroups exist and how to align them as a positive force for the environment and as a force for promoting the capacity of the environment in its "healing" mission.

Determinants of culture in a Behavioral Health System of Care

Given the importance of culture in a Behavioral Health System of Care, we identify three key determinants needed to shape and grow culture. They include how leadership articulates and embraces the healing mission, how the organization fosters critical values in the workplace. and how the organization takes care of its employees.

The mission is alive

Behavioral health, for a variety of reasons, is a field that people tend to choose to go into more than accidentally find themselves in. In fact, we would say that people choose to enter the field for deeply personal reasons, some of which they are aware of, and some that they learn about through their work. Most enter the field, at least in part, because they want to "help" others and perhaps different from other areas of healthcare, because they want to be engaged in meaningful relationships with the people they are helping.

They also do this knowing at the outset, or quickly realizing after beginning in the field, that financial compensation for their work will, perhaps (hopefully), be "OK" as in fair to good but certainly not excellent or superior to what they will see their counterparts earning in other fields. What most employees expect to get in return is the opportunity to do the meaningful work they set out to do and to work alongside people who are there for similar reasons. Most are looking for an environment that values their efforts and takes its healing mission seriously. This "alignment" of an employee's work effort with their colleagues and how that meshes with the organization as a whole is central to their personal value proposition. It impacts their motivation and willingness to accept limitations in compensation, benefits, and working conditions for the opportunity to work in a field and organization that mirrors their values.

Understanding this connection between staff members and the mission of the organization is, of course, an important starting point for leadership in its efforts to shape culture, but it really is just that – a starting point. There are very few healthcare organizations of any kind that do not see themselves as healers and use compelling words beautifully to communicate that effect in their mission statements. However, it is how the mission is embraced and practiced daily, how it is kept alive, that is the critical variable that determines the organizational culture. And it is what separates highly successful organizations from others. This is the number one job of leadership.

Leadership provides the focus and insistence of the organization's culture through *continuous intentional action and communication* about the healing mission of the organization and the people (the entire staff) who work in the organization. This is accomplished through personal modeling, by identifying important values and contributions of its members, and by carefully balancing the business and administrative needs of the organization with the healing mission.

This is a huge task and the essence of making a healing culture come alive. The CEO or President and other senior leaders set the tone for the entire organization. If the CEO "walks the walk" and can be seen as actively engaged and modeling the importance of the healing culture in word and deed, other senior leaders will follow, and soon these actions will spread throughout the organization. But if the CEO determines that he or she is too busy for these activities and is focused completely on the business side of the organization and external matters and delegates these duties to Human Resources or other departments, the organizational culture is doomed. It will be weak and unevenly spread, subgroups will develop their own cultures (often negative) and, over time, these subgroups will clash with each other.

Example

A mission-driven Behavioral Health System of Care will have many ways of communicating the importance and appreciation of its work to its employees. At one point in its development, Walden Behavioral Care was looking for a way to recognize the everyday, often unrecognized acts, of "doing good" by its staff at all levels of the organization. We wanted to highlight acts that went under the radar so formulated what we call the "Spot" award. The Spot award embraced the idea that any staff member could recognize a co-worker at any time by "catching them on the spot" and filling out a very short form which cited the worker and their contribution. The Spot award encouraged people to look for ways in which co-workers quietly furthered the organization's stated mission and values through their efforts on behalf of patients or other staff.

Once the form was submitted, the acknowledgments were "seconded" by a supervisor and sent to HR for distribution to the senior staff, including the CEO. An email was sent out to the entire organization identifying the awardee and highlighting their great work and commitment to the values we share. The fun part was the onslaught of congratulatory notes that the awardee would receive from other staff and senior leaders. Each email, from across the organization, would typically thank the employee for their service and most importantly for the actions they took to further the mission and values of the organization.

Balancing the clinical and business missions

One of the most difficult things for the CEO and other senior leaders to do is balance the business mission of the organization with the healing mission. We have discussed this task in our chapter on Leadership, but it deserves mention again because of its importance and centrality to the issue of culture. Some see these as diametrically opposed. Clinicians in a Behavioral Health System of Care are very attuned to it and tend to be acutely aware of their workload and are especially sensitive to the pressure they feel when they experience a change in the volume of cases they are holding.

When a time of increased volume occurs, clinicians may perceive and voice concerns that they are unable to provide the quality of service they would like. They will cite the quantity of work they are being asked to do and the potential impact to the quality of care they offer. For some, there will be suspicion of the pressures of the business side of the equation and feeling the need to spread themselves thinly and the impact of the decreased time spent directly engaging with patients. All of these take away from the meaningful interaction that facilitates healing and recovery.

For the organization, this experience of a wave of "high volume" can occur at often unanticipated times and with little opportunity for adequate planning. It can result from a variety of forces which impact the workforce such as staff absences due to sickness or family leave (i.e. maternity leave, etc.), unfilled positions, actual changes (increases) in service demand, and budgetary cutbacks. Regardless of the reason, when staff experience a gap between what they desire to do in providing a professional healing service with the demands that arise because of immediate business conditions and day-to-day ratio of staff to patients, they begin to question the true intentions of the organization. They may even doubt its commitment to living up to its mission. If this becomes a chronic concern of staff, morale will undoubtedly suffer, and the organizational culture of healing cannot be sustained. When these conditions continue for longer periods of time, employees grow resentful and tend to "vote with their feet," meaning they leave to work elsewhere where they perceive that there is a better balance and firmer commitment to the healing mission.

We strongly advise that leaders in a Behavioral Health System of Care, from the CEO down to program directors and supervisors, address issues of workforce openly and frequently, both in terms of general trends in the industry and regarding specific concerns voiced by staff. This sort of communication begins with some education about how staff budgets are developed and how workforce decisions are made. We want staff to be aware of the factors that impact the day-to-day staffing complements as well as target caseloads.

Our experience has taught us that staff are far more willing to give management "the benefit of the doubt" in terms of their intentions in upholding the importance of the healing environment when they are more transparent in their communication about these central issues. Among the most important pieces of information that can be shared is a rudimentary understanding of the mechanics of budgeting – specifically, that staff budgets are built to the expected "average caseload," and factors that may cause this to vary from time to time. On many occasions, we have observed aloud for staff consumption that "management is highly sensitive to low census (volume) and staff is highly sensitive to high census which is why budgets are built to the expected average."

If these annual assumptions about volume prove to be wrong, the staffing complement is changed, but only after some sustained experience, usually not less than a fiscal quarter year or three-month period. With this background knowledge, staff are better equipped and hence more likely to cope effectively with temporary high-volume periods. Additional efforts by management to recognize and assist with caseload peaks (i.e. recruiting additional temporary staff or additional clerical support, offering to re-assign a staff member from one location to another, etc.) can greatly ease the situation and maintain integrity in the healing mission.

Case example

Anticipating staffing needs for a child psychiatry unit based on census is a challenging task. We had learned over the years that we could anticipate a census dip in the summer months and then a quick pick up once school resumes in September. Of course, most people want full-time jobs, and it is hard to find people who can work only selected months, leaving us with a budgetary challenge; how to get through a period of low census and then to manage the rapid increase in census without precipitating a staffing crisis.

We thought we were in a good place one year when we had several staff members unexpectedly asking for the summer off. Some had childcare needs and others wanted extended time off for travel. With the full expectation that our census would follow its predictable pattern, we agreed to all the requests. We felt assured that in September, our numbers would rebound, and we would then be back to our full complement of staff, each member refreshed from their time off. Of course, in an inpatient psychiatry program, things don't always go according to plan. In fact, that year, rather than the predicted slower pace with a low census for the summer months, for reasons we still don't understand, the exact opposite happened. The census ballooned.

On the good side, we had the highest census quarter of the year, which greatly relieved some of our budgetary shortfalls. But on the downside, we struggled throughout the summer to maintain adequate staffing. And, of course, throughout the first few weeks of the summer, there was a palpable rise in discontent among the ranks. Many staff members were furious at what they saw as the business interests of the organization overriding a staffing crisis. Almost everyone was being asked to work overtime and, in some cases, people were mandated to cover shifts. Tensions rose with the summer heat with many seeing it as a black-and-white issue of profits over quality healthcare.

Increasingly aware of how upset the staff were, we convened a meeting with the entire staff. After carefully listening to their concerns, we reminded everyone of how we had carefully planned for the summer with the good intention of managing our staffing according to what history had taught us. We acknowledged that things certainly didn't turn out the way we intended and asked them directly to give their managers the benefit of a doubt. We assured them that our current situation was not something that we could have anticipated nor frankly wanted.

The group seemed to shift with the honesty of the discussion, especially the reassurance that our situation was the unintended result of what we thought was careful planning. We then told everyone that we would continue to look for additional short-term staff to help for the rest of the summer, and that we were actively working on a plan to pull some staff members from another program in the system to assist. We, of course, let everyone know that we would continue to compensate people at an overtime rate for the shifts that they picked up. And lastly, we asked people to work together through this difficult time and reminded everyone that this crisis would be time limited. We promised to get through it together.

Cultural values

Most healthcare organizations espouse similar values even if they use different words to describe them. These values are frequently articulated alongside the mission and speak to an organizational dedication of caring and compassion for the patients that they treat. And a second tier of values that most healthcare organizations aspire to relates to the quality of services provided: a high degree of professionalism, a concern for safety, and a commitment to excellent outcomes. It would be highly unusual for a healthcare organization to <u>not</u> include statements about these ideals in their organizational documents, employee handbooks, and marketing materials, and we can all agree that these are worthy aspirations. However, these statements are mere marketing strategies and have limited actual impact unless there is a continual and intentional effort on the part of management to communicate and engage in actual workplace practices that highlight and support the expression of values-oriented behavior.

We repeat our key understanding of healthcare organizational culture: what the patient ultimately feels about the services provided by the organization is a by-product of the workplace culture. In practice, this means that how well the staff do in living up to the aspirations and articulations of the mission and values of the organization is largely dependent on how the staff feel they themselves and their co-workers are resourced and treated by the organization. The attitudes and beliefs of the employees of the organization relative to their daily existence and working conditions are at the core of workplace culture. This is especially true in behavioral healthcare where staff members often experience a sense of deprivation.

Culture builders

In our experience, the things that seem to make the most difference to employees working in behavioral healthcare settings that support the ongoing positive functioning of workplace culture are:

- Fairness and opportunity
- Inclusion and respect
- Supervision and training
- Collegiality and community engagement

Fairness and opportunity

Individuals who make the decision to work in the behavioral health field understand early on that monetary compensation may be limited and certainly should not be a driving force in their career planning. However, in accepting this general condition, the behavioral health workforce is extremely sensitive when it comes to compensation. If they feel they are not being treated fairly within the cohort of their peers and not afforded equal access to opportunities to improve their compensation and role when promotion opportunities become available, dissatisfaction can escalate quickly. This may not be all that different from any work environment, but there is an added component at play here because these employees truly expect that their supervisors and managers understand that at some level, they have made a sacrifice to work in the field. It is critical that employees trust that their supervisors or managers in the organization are looking out for them and their interests to the best of their ability. This means that each employee believes there is genuine effort to compensate them fairly when compared to others and to support opportunities for advancement when they become available within the organization. When situations arise in which fairness or opportunity is at question, it is damaging to this unspoken compact between the employee and the organization.

Financial compensation is only one of the numerous areas in which fairness and opportunity are at stake. Tools and resources (i.e. computers, phones), work schedules and assignments, office space, training opportunities, social events, and access to advancement are also closely watched. This often also has to do with a perception of scarcity by the employee and a feeling that if you miss one opportunity, it will be a long time before another presents itself.

Example

Jim, a young mental health counselor with a Bachelors in Sociology and little over a year of experience in the field, approached his supervisor, Joe, who oversaw the entire pool of Mental Health Counselors at a hundred-bed psychiatric hospital. Joe could tell right away that Jim was worked up and thought it probably had to do with the demands of the weekend, maybe staffing or some other problem with a particularly difficult patient. But, on this occasion, it was far more personal. With emotion in his voice, Jim told Joe that he was upset because in conversation over the weekend he had learned that a newly hired Mental Health Counselor, someone he was charged with training, had been hired at almost $2.00 per hour: more than Jim was currently making. Jim said he was so surprised that he did a small survey of his colleagues and found many inconsistencies in pay among his peers. He demanded an immediate adjustment to his compensation which Joe was not authorized to make. Joe told him that he would research the issue and get back to him.

Joe was not completely unaware of this issue. Part of his job had grown much more difficult in the wake of the Covid pandemic as he was charged with finding enough staff to fill the shifts. At times, it was an almost impossible task, and at times, the hospital was forced to pay rates well above what had been budgeted. Joe brought the issue to senior management and the Human Resources Department was asked to conduct a review of all employees by job category. The results quickly confirmed that there were discrepancies and similar disparities in almost all job functions. Some of the salary differences were striking and unlike generations in the past, how much one makes is no longer a private matter, rather a frequent topic of conversation. And with Jim's discovery, it was likely to spread as a much wider issue.

As the scope of the problem grew and the price tag for correcting the inequity escalated, the impact on the entire organization was clear. It was decided that the solution had to be addressed in the next budget cycle and the process slowed down. As days became weeks, Jim recruited other Mental Health Counselors to his cause and as a group demanded to meet with the Vice President of Human Resources. They were angry and complained about the unfair treatment. Eventually, pay adjustments were made, but the morale of the Mental Health Counselors as a group suffered with many complaining that they felt like they were second-class citizens.

Inclusion and respect

This category covers two related meanings. The first is strictly work related and refers to the idea that staff in behavioral health organizations, especially clinical staff, expect to have the opportunity to contribute to the treatment of individuals that they work with. This occurs through both electronic and direct communication with the clinical leaders within any treatment environment. In many places, this occurs through the process of treatment team where staff gather as professionals to consider the course of treatment and make plans and decisions regarding care. Expectations around providing input relative to individual patients varies (and should vary), but the "TEAM" works best when there is a willingness on the part of the leaders to consider all the data and views of staff that are working actively with the patient.

This can be difficult with very complex cases, although that is usually the time when the input of multiple sources is most helpful. Programs that operate twenty-four hours per day are some of the best examples as patient behavior may vary quite broadly from day to night to weekend. It is often the staff that works nights and weekends that "feels left out" and least included in the planning around treatment. It is often those same staff that are on hand to work most directly with challenging behavioral and psychiatric symptoms.

A second meaning of inclusion and respect refers to the degree of comfort and acceptance of the work environment for individuals from underrepresented segments of the population, including ethnic minority groups and individuals identifying as members of the LGBTQ+ community. In promoting a healing environment for patients, stigma and other forms of "micro-aggression" must be directly addressed. Staff members working in behavioral health environments expect to be able to work comfortably within their chosen identity and expect the support of the organization.

Example

As part of a growing movement in behavioral health, a large hospital decided to add people with lived experience to their staffing model. These are individuals who have struggled in their own lives with a mental illness and now in recovery have a perspective to offer both staff and patients. In theory, the current staff at the hospital thought of the idea as progressive and said they were open to it. It did not, however, work out that way. The individual who was hired felt distanced almost immediately. From their perspective, they were marginalized and although they were part of staff meetings and treatment teams, felt as though their contributions were minimized.

After just two months of employment, the individual with lived experience felt isolated and ineffective and went to the hospital administrator to resign.

Unaware of the individual's experience, the administrator was taken aback. From her perspective, this had been a step forward in addressing stigma and she was disheartened to hear that the idea in practice was not embraced by all her staff. So, she made a bold move. She convinced her employee with lived experience not to leave. She restated her commitment to employing individuals with lived experience, and importantly, committed to hiring others with lived experience. She expressed a genuine sense of hope that with more of a presence in the hospital the risk of isolation would decrease, and the value of a lived experience perspective would grow.

Supervision and training

In a job interview, we always talk about an organizational culture of learning. We talk about the culture of learning that we have developed in our organization and invite an applicant to join us in a search for better, more effective treatments. It's an important invitation and part of what we want to communicate is the message that we are all contributors to our collective learning and that as an organization, we are always learning. It speaks to an important part of our culture.

Part of this learning culture is a commitment to provide regular and consistent supervision and ongoing training opportunities. In truth, many behavioral health organizations take this lightly. Supervision, when it happens, is spotty and rushed with the employee often feeling like they are imposing on their supervisor for their time. It is common for formal training to be the responsibility of the employee on one's own time and at their expense.

We make a commitment to an employee to provide a qualified supervisor and the time needed for weekly supervision. We expect that supervisors within the organization will approach this task with the seriousness it requires, scheduling meetings in advance and every week. Sessions are used to cover the basic tasks of the supervisee's role as well as an opportunity for thoughtful discussion about clinical problem areas and even one's work environment. In our experience, most employees value this time tremendously. They see that their growth as a clinician is enhanced by the time spent discussing their clinical work with someone more senior.

Since some clinicians join us at the beginning phase of their career when weekly supervision by a licensed provider is required by their board as they work toward a higher level of licensure. For them, our commitment to providing supervision becomes a significant benefit of their employment. It is also an essential part of orienting each clinician and a concrete sign of our investment in their clinical growth.

The same is true with ongoing training. If the culture of the organization values learning, then high-quality training opportunities are a critical opportunity for employees to learn about behavioral health topics often in a shared forum. In addition to a monthly Grand Rounds speaker series on a range of topics suggested by our staff, we have always kept a budget to support attendance at local and regional conferences, and dollars for tuition reimbursement for coursework that relates to a person's job function.

Collegiality and engagement

There are numerous "offsetting rewards" that individuals working in this field expect as part of their value proposition when they choose behavioral health. Among the most important is the opportunity to work alongside like-minded, caring, compassionate people and to be able to enjoy their collegiality both formally and informally at work. These relationships are important and are usually the way that individual staff first connect to the organization. That is, they connect first to co-workers and then hopefully to the organization and its mission and values. There is an expectation that the work environment will support this type of collegial interaction in the form of case reviews, supervision, training, and various team building activities and it is critical that local managers nurture these team environments as building blocks for the greater system as well.

Case example

The husband of a senior manager works in the hospitality industry, and we learned from her that in that industry employees are trained to greet people. Staff members of all ranks are trained in orientation to say hello by name to all staff members they encounter throughout the day. And if an employee encounters a guest who might look lost, employees are trained to approach the guest in a friendly manner and to ask if there is anything that they can do to help. It seems like a powerful way to build a welcoming culture and to foster connections among team members.

Our acute care unit was already a friendly group, so we chose to focus directly on approaching a visitor and asking if they needed help. We challenged our staff to approach any guest or visitor to the unit who might appear to be lost or waiting in one of our waiting areas. We asked our employees to approach the visitor in a welcoming manner and to ask if they had been helped. If there was something that they needed, we empowered our staff to attempt to solve the problem, not needing to check with a supervisor.

We used our usual forms of communication to get people on board with the practice, but by far, the biggest training effect was in role modeling by key leaders. It was a powerful intervention when all the managers in our organization started to approach visitors and offered to help, it quickly caught on and became part of our culture. Many of our staff later commented that the simple act made them feel as though they had some ownership in the program, and we got a lot of feedback from visitors that we were a friendly and helpful place. Many referenced that they had been approached, sometimes by more than one staff member, all of whom genuinely wanted to be helpful.

We have also observed that staff in behavioral health expect their organizations to be engaged and positive contributors to the world around them. They want to feel comfortable that the organization they work for is a "good" place that gives back to the community at large, and they want to be able to participate with their colleagues in activities that make them "feel good" about themselves and their organization.

Management retreat

As an organization, we created an annual management retreat for all mid- and upper-level managers. This event brought together our leadership from all disciplines and across the system for a two-day event filled with inspirational talks, educational seminars, and social activities. The agenda was developed with input from the entire list of attendees, with the intention of deepening the group's connection to the organizational mission and to each other. Each retreat had a core theme or message that was important to the organization and the day always included some sort of "state of the state" address by the CEO and other C-suite executives, stimulating talks by internal experts and invited guests and plenty of time for socializing and having fun together. These retreats were important in that they served as both an opportunity to review the past year(s) and look to the future as well as express gratitude to all the attendees for their efforts on behalf of the organization.

Example

It had been a challenging year with the growth of new programs that stretched the geography of the organization. Now, with more employees and a growing regional reach, there was the perception that what was once a small group of people who knew each other well had grown with many new faces and less connection. In preparation for the retreat, we worked to develop an agenda that would give everyone a sense of ownership in the company.

We met as a group to plan the day and how to create a sense of ownership, when one of our program directors spoke up and told a story about working in a prior job at a well-known golf club. She said the club, which was known for its pristine course and grounds, had institutionalized a sense of pride in the appearance of the club. There were many ways this was communicated among the employees, but one she said that really stuck out in her mind was quite simply, that everyone on the staff picked up litter. That meant that everyone, even the president of the club. If you were driving a golf cart around and saw candy wrapper by the side on the grass, it was part of the culture to pull over, get out of the cart, and pick up the wrapper. She said everyone did it and with something so simple came a belief that everyone was responsible for the course. Implied in that was that no one was above doing a simple task to make the club more presentable. Everyone had ownership.

Our agenda planning meeting then had a robust discussion about pride and ownership of our organization. We decided to use the candy wrapper as a symbol of pride and ownership, and we built an agenda around the themes of pride in our work and a shared responsibility for our success as an organization. Activities and round table discussions were planned to further develop the idea and to challenge the leadership group to identify their own small tasks that would distinguish our culture from any other health organization. When the big day arrived, at each participant's place at a table was a gift of a small ceramic candy wrapper.

Communicating value and appreciation for every job category

The importance of this is probably not distinct for a Behavioral Health System of Care as compared to other types of healthcare organization, or really any other type of company, but we find it extremely important, nonetheless. What perhaps makes it more important in this situation is the objective of creating a "healing environment." To truly create a healing environment requires the building of a healthy culture, and this is certainly enhanced when the people working in the organization feel that their work is valued and appreciated. Communicating respect and value is, however, a big issue in the field of behavioral health because of the issue of stigma which affects our patients on a day-to-day basis. So, even as we work to remove stigma from our treatment environments, it is incumbent upon us to treat our fellow colleagues at all levels and all types of jobs with respect.

In a Behavioral Health System of Care, there may be numerous groups of employees who are at risk of feeling disrespected or marginalized. One group that is often at risk is the line level mental health aides (variously referred to as counselors, recovery coaches, etc.). These are the individuals who work most closely with patients throughout the days and evenings, weekends, and holidays. They are the people who are directly "in the line of fire" when patients become dysregulated and are responsible for managing crisis situations. They are often the lowest compensated employees too, and while there are benefits to doing the job, especially if they are intending to progress in the field, they do not receive the respect and appreciation from the patients in the same way as the physicians and psychologists and other professional staff do.

It is critical for the organization to communicate true respect and appreciation to this group, and this can be done in a variety of ways, including awards and recognition, special training opportunities, dedicated supervision, and opportunities for advancement to "lead" mental health counselor. Additionally, direct communication from the organization's management and clinical leaders in each program to recognize work done well is essential.

Another group to be concerned about are those company employees in administrative support roles, individuals who are not part of the mainstream clinical activity. While they are not involved in the clinical activity per se, many of these individuals come into contact with patients and loved ones in a variety of ways, including billing and collections activity, phone and facility reception, admissions, facility cleaning and maintenance, food service, and other activities. Patients and families, referral sources, and insurance representatives do not distinguish among staff when interacting with an organization; they form opinions and have reactions according to their perception as to how they have been treated by whoever they speak with. It is extremely important that non-clinical employees participate in the company culture just as the clinical staff do. In fact, many of them have elected to be employed by the organization because of its healing mission and need to know that their efforts contribute to a greater good.

References

Deci, E. L. and Ryan, R. M. (1985). *Intrinsic Motivation and Self-Determination in Human Behavior*. Plenum Press.

Parsons, T. (1951). *The Social System*. Free Press.

Schein, E. H. (2010). *Organizational Culture and Leadership*, 4th Edition. Jossey-Bass.

8

LEADING A BEHAVIORAL HEALTH SYSTEM OF CARE

Behavioral health organizations play a crucial role in providing essential mental health and substance abuse services to individuals worldwide. Within these organizations, effective leadership is paramount for ensuring the delivery of high-quality care, fostering innovation, and navigating complex regulatory landscapes (Cliff 2012). Effective leadership sets the strategic direction and vision for the organization, ensuring alignment with its mission to provide accessible, effective, and compassionate care to individuals in need. Additionally, effective leadership fosters a culture of excellence, innovation, and continuous improvement, driving positive outcomes for both patients and staff members.

Key positions include the Chief Executive Officer (CEO), who is responsible for overall strategic leadership and management of the organization and oversees the development and implementation of strategies to meet improvement goals and initiatives aimed at achieving the organization's mission and goals (Zimring et al. 2008). The Chief Medical Officer (CMO) provides formal clinical leadership and oversight, ensuring the delivery of high-quality, evidence-based care as well as playing a key role in improving the quality of care and sustainability of healthcare (Berghout et al. 2017). The Chief Financial Officer (CFO) is responsible for financial management, budgeting, financial reporting, compliance, and risk management and is increasingly being asked to bring innovative ideas to the table while ensuring the organization's fiscal health and sustainability (O'Brien 2008). And the Chief Clinical Officer (CCO) who oversees clinical operations, ensuring the delivery of safe, effective, patient-centered care through collaboration with interdisciplinary teams. The CCO also

DOI: 10.4324/9781315177366-9

monitors clinical outcomes, quality metrics, and patient satisfaction to drive continuous improvement.

Everyone working in behavioral health can quickly recount both the worst and the very best leaders they have worked with. They will tell you compelling stories of working with bad leaders, sometimes wondering why these individuals even worked in the field and many will express a profound sense of disappointment with leadership in general. They may point to a huge disconnect between what they expected versus what they experienced in the mission of the organization and cite how leadership seemed to unapologetically operate outside of that. Many will talk about missing a sense of inspiration from leadership with an emerging theme in which money and business were seen as the primary drivers with little appreciation for the science and art of behavioral health. We have found that behavioral health providers are hungry for strong leadership. They crave working for individuals who understand the deep emotional connection people experience in the field and desperately look for someone that can inspire them to do their best in their everyday work with a sense of hope for the future.

While leadership is important in any endeavor, it is a critical part in the success of a Behavioral Health System of Care. And while leaders come in all varieties and certainly each with their own distinctive style, there are certain key qualities that leaders in a Behavioral Health System of Care must possess for the system to operate effectively, efficiently, and with a deep sense of humanity. This is the subject discussed here. We support a leadership model that distributes authority, within limits, to a group of some fifteen to thirty individuals. It is important that these individuals meet regularly and function as a unit – a TEAM – which can operate a good size Behavioral Health System of Care with multiple levels of care, many locations, and operating budgets approaching $1B or more.

Distributed authority

This is a key concept. Distributed leadership empowers leaders in the organization to essentially "run a business." They are permitted to make decisions, especially day-to-day clinical and operating decisions, without extensive consultation with others. For it to work, there must be a high degree of trust from the CEO and other C-suite executives who work to ensure that decisions are consistent with the basic values and mission of the organization. Oversight essentially means making sure that these empowered decision makers adhere to the organization's operating parameters regarding critical functions, especially spending. Most organizations seek the optimal balance between centralized and local authority, but the complexity and sheer number of decisions that are required on a day-to-day basis for any component of a Behavioral Health System of Care makes it necessary to embrace and foster a distributed leadership model.

Distributed leadership has many advantages. For the program or component of a system of care, the distributed leadership model creates efficiency and focus. Individuals in leadership roles within a program or sub-component of a Behavioral Health System of Care are responsible for shaping general operating procedures to the local environment and developing staff resources that best fit the specific needs of that program (business). These become more and more refined over time especially if there is continuity in leadership.

Additionally, healthcare businesses often have formal oversight bodies at both the state and local level. It is imperative that delegated leaders be knowledgeable about the regulations in place for each level of care and responsive to these requirements in addition to the "rules and regulations" that are part of the organization's operating culture. When local leadership is strong and successful in responding to the needs of the organization and the oversight authorities and when the entity can run at a high volume and meets its clinical and regulatory obligations, things can start to happen. It allows the larger system to take on additional challenges and expand because the central authority, the CEO, and senior team can turn their attention elsewhere.

For the local leader, distributed authority allows for a sense of autonomy and entrepreneurship. Individuals in these roles certainly support and meet the requirements of the organization but also have latitude to solve problems, support staff, and plan future projects. These activities are self-reinforcing and can in turn lead to higher retention of talented individuals. Local leaders who run components of a system, often small businesses themselves with $1M in revenue or more, develop a sense of mastery and ownership. They, and their direct reports, tend to invest fully in the work of the enterprise and take great pride in their successes. The skills and expertise in management that they learn make them strong candidates for higher level jobs as they become available. We discuss this more later in the chapter.

More than anything else, leaders in a Behavioral Health System of Care provide three things: they uphold the values of the organization, they nurture its culture, and they aggressively support the system to function as a system. This definition applies to all leaders at all levels of the organization but, most critically, to the few people at the top, especially the CEO (Chief Executive Officer), the most senior physician (Chief Medical Officer), and the most senior clinicians (Chief Clinical Officer, Chief Nursing Officer). The central importance of these individuals comes from their scope of authority and the fact that others in the organization will look to them for guidance as to how they should carry out their duties and will most likely follow their lead. It is important that they be consistent in word and action as they are constantly being watched as models or, in the negative case, to see what types of behaviors they are discouraging. Given their importance, we will spend some time on each.

Chief Executive Officer

The Chief Executive Officer (CEO) is the most critical leadership figure in a Behavioral Health System of Care. In most organizations, this person is often seen as having an external focus or responsibility, often being the face of the organization to the public and key constituents. They are also the ones in the organization that can anticipate trends in the environment and appropriately position the enterprise for future success. In a Behavioral Health System of Care, the role of the CEO is more expansive. Certainly, they are the external face of the organization, but more importantly, they must create a strong presence within the organization. There, they are the system's tone setter, chief advocate of the mission and its people and, when needed, the upholder and even enforcer of the key operating principles of the system. While not all Behavioral Health Systems of Care are successful even with a strong CEO, it is certain that without this pivotal role, the system will not be successful and may never truly meet its potential.

While there are many qualities that are attributed to an ideal of leadership, the truth is that many highly effective CEOs can employ a wide variety of styles. There is no template or set standard. With that being said, we believe that there are some qualities which a CEO in a Behavioral Health System of Care must possess. The most significant of these is that the CEO must truly enjoy people and appreciate knowing them in a personal way. Specifically, they must enjoy connecting with people in the organization, not through an affable ability to simply remember names, but as a genuine individual who possesses a sincere interest in knowing employees as people even in their lives outside of the organization. It is about creating a feeling of true concern for a person's well-being, their family, and their growth within the field. If a CEO can connect and communicate in this way, he or she can inspire employees to fully commit to the mission of the organization and ultimately to do their best work.

This ability to connect with employees is critical to the building of an organization's culture and directly relates to the longevity of the workforce. Most health organizations struggle with rapidly cycling providers, employees who "stop by" for a brief stint all the while looking for their next best deal. A strong organization needs a core of individuals who hold the culture and are satisfied with where they work. These are the people who are committed to the organization and are invested in who is joining as the next generation of providers and leaders, how people are trained, and how they will be positioned for the future of the organization. Creating this core and maintaining it is part of the tone and culture set by the CEO.

We spoke earlier about the importance of the CEO believing firmly in the value of a system of care and having an intuitive commitment to making it effectively work. This unyielding belief in a system of care and the relentless pursuit of its working is a central piece of how a successful CEO thinks and makes decisions. He or she will be faced with multiple challenges every day that can have a significant impact on the system and each decision is watched by many. When decisions are consciously and consistently made in the interest of the system, it counteracts the almost natural tendency for people to make exceptions and veer away toward more familiar structures. A CEO must be steadfast in their belief and actions.

Like a parent with many children, the CEO is the key person internally who spreads the "love" among the many sub-components of a system of care. Importantly, they never choose a favorite. The CEO must give due credit and attention to each program and department when they demonstrate individual accomplishments and cooperative system engagement. And while employees who directly interface with patients and their families are recognized, it is especially important for the CEO to openly acknowledge the contributions of the organization's administrative functions. These are employees often not involved in the day-to-day clinical activity who can easily become disengaged from the mainstream mission.

Every Behavioral Health System of Care is a business, often a big business. If the business slows and becomes inefficient, the consequences are felt all over the system. Understanding the importance of what happens behind the scenes to ensure cash flow, recruitment, hiring and taking care of staff, and conducting the marketing and communications functions is as critical as any treatment intervention that a patient receives. A wise CEO shines light on this work and amplifies the importance of those administrative functions as they allow the clinical talent to thrive.

Second, the CEO is the chief communicator to all parts of a system of the key components related to organizational mission. As a behavioral health organization, the enterprise is often so focused on its clinical mission that it is easy to forget about the business mission, but this would be a mistake. Why? Because any enterprise that forgets about the importance of the business mission of operating well clearly puts the other mission, the clinical mission, at great risk.

It is frequently the case that people who work in behavioral health, namely clinicians and other healthcare providers, are not interested in business. They often chose this field because of their interest in working as helpers with people and see business as almost the antithesis of this. We believe to make the system vibrant; it is important to keep business front and center, not something to be shied away from. And as such, it is important for the CEO and other leaders in the organization to keep the importance of operating a strong business very firmly in mind for all employees. One way this idea can be framed for them is this: "the clinical mission and business mission of this organization are co-equal; one without the other makes the organization doomed to fail." This statement is easy to make and has worked well in communicating the reliance that each mission has on the other. We like the positive framing just as well: "a strong clinical mission is why people come here to get care; a strong business allows us to take care of our staff and continue to grow."

Lastly, the CEO plays a central role in making sure that the components of the system behave according to the system's operating principles. This must begin with a firm belief on the part of the CEO that a system of care is the best option for providing treatment. He or she must then communicate this often and clearly throughout the organization. Much of this effort should be accomplished by other leaders in the system, those who report directly to the CEO and others down the chain of command, but in the event of a challenge to the logic of working the system, for instance with a highly complex or high-profile case, the CEO must get involved and make decisions that ultimately support the system of care though they may be unpopular to one program or another. In relation to decisions that have clinical complexity, the CEO will usually defer to the CMO and CCO to make the decision after due consideration of the clinical issues involved. This maintains credibility in the clinical mission as most staff just want their input to be heard and understand that "perfect" answers are not to be had in many of these situations. As long as there has been a serious review of issues and concerns, they are likely to accept whatever the outcome is.

It is critical for all C-suite executives, vice presidents, program directors, and other managers to be in synch with the CEO and for the CEO to communicate clearly to these leaders. In a Behavioral Health System of Care, each leader has a "constituency" of individuals who work under their guidance, so it is important that each leader understand and endorse the mission, values, and operating principles of the Behavioral Health System of Care. We have found it essential to have regularly scheduled meetings with the CEO and C-suite executives which reinforce the strategic direction and operating principles of the system. Like any other type of organization, accountability is crucial, and the CEO plays the major role in this area.

We are also supporters of encouraging broad input from leaders in developing strategy and direction, including annual budgets. Many come to the table with "wish lists" for their programs or division, all of which are usually good ideas, but understand that once established, these plans will require performance in meeting revenue targets. Specific reminders and reinforcing conversations with the CEO and C-suite executives if there is slippage in performance is often necessary. This can be done in many ways. We have had success with a "benevolent dictator" approach. These conversations, which often focus on revenue, should take place organically in routine meetings and settings where performance is being reviewed. Conflict avoidance is not a good trait for a CEO to have as it is never a good idea to avoid calling attention to real or potential issues, in fact, the sooner the better.

Regularly scheduled leadership meetings are critically important for the CEO to create a sense of presence and to communicate important issues in the organization, but their true value is in creating a sense of team among the leaders present. Not only do these programs or sub-components of the system need to operate in synch with the CEO, but they also need to operate in synch with each other. We have found that developing this sense can be a more difficult task as many programs may not share the same day-to-day challenges. However, in a broader sense, these regular meetings reinforce the notion of "system-ness," which can focus on the entirety of resources that the system can bring to bear in support of our patients. It is important for local leaders to consistently be reminded that they are a part of a larger whole and that each component is essential in the working of the system. When a sense of team is created, these leaders can operate in a complementary fashion, share information easily, and understand their unique contributions to the clinical enterprise. This is the fuel that makes the system perform at its best.

Of note, we have leaders of non-clinical functions in the organization also attend these meetings. And the goal is similar – to reinforce the idea that the system is more than a local program and that collaboration with all parts is essential to operating a successful system. The CEO's role in these meetings is often like a sports or performance coach: part cheerleader, part educator, part therapist. Most of all, the CEO wants to acknowledge individual and team success in its many forms, identify areas of improvement, and exhort the team to aspire to and achieve better outcomes for patients and families.

We have developed some practices and focus areas that we have found to be helpful and important in carrying out the CEO duties. These practices impact organizational "ambience," shape the way communication flows and the way in which individuals can connect to the organization. At the base of each of these practices is an understanding that people do not actually connect to an organization; they mostly connect to other people in the organization, and the more, the better. This is probably true for any organization, but we think this is especially important for individuals who choose to work in the field of mental health.

CEO practices that enhance organizational "ambience"

Open-door policy

Over the years, we have endorsed an "open-door" policy for communicating with leadership from the top down. What this means is that anyone in the company is free to speak or communicate directly with the CEO. This practice sends a powerful message – everyone from top to bottom is important and has the "right" to speak up and have input. New employees are often disbelieving. "It's just lip service," they say, and, in truth, there are those who will not take advantage of it. But many do. This practice established by the CEO, is an open invitation to all employees and sets a precedent that all leaders are obligated to follow. We have found that it creates more robust back-and-forth communication between leadership at different levels and their staff.

Leaders trained in other organizations are not always comfortable with the "open-door" policy. It is rarely what they are used to with many coming from a hierarchical structure in which someone "lower" in the organization would never "go over the head of their boss" and speak directly to the CEO. Some have a fear that any information shared by an employee to the CEO may cast their direct supervisor in a negative light. However, we have found that often, an open-door policy leads to more open communication with managers and leaders at each level and a similar openness between leaders and their own boss. Leaders throughout the organization learn to communicate about issues earlier and more directly to their boss because it is far better to raise these concerns themselves than it is for their boss to hear about them from others, especially aggrieved parties.

This direct communication can take many forms in addition to face-to-face meetings, including individual phone contact, emails, intranet messaging, and other communications apps and group settings such as all company meetings and visits by the CEO to individual programs or departments. Each CEO can decide as to the specific channels he or she prefers, and the amount of time set aside for this activity. Often, the CEO charges his/her administrative assistant to assist in structuring the interaction by getting some brief information about the agenda and then scheduling the interaction. The CEO may also request that the assistant gather additional information prior to the connection to make the time most useful.

Example

An employee with ten years of service as a middle manager called recently to tell the CEO that he was leaving the organization. As he relayed the information, he spoke warmly about his time at the organization and regretfully about leaving now that his life situation (two young children) and a long commute made it impossible to continue. He stated that he stayed much longer than he originally anticipated and attributed his interest in the organization to a discussion that he had with the CEO and some other leaders early in his career when "I didn't think I was even on the radar." He went on to say that "I was so impressed that the

CEO took time to speak and follow-up with me" that I just knew this was a great place to work and my feelings never changed afterwards.

Example

A CEO in a competitor organization was recalling past decisions, some in which he felt a sense of pride and others some regret. He ran a very hierarchical organization with each layer contributing to the final product. When asked about the regrets over the years, he sadly recalled a great working relationship he had shared with a former COO. Unfortunately, her performance had started to slip at a crucial time for the company and he made the decision, somewhat abruptly, to move her out of the organization. He recalled telling her and while she was clearly upset, she acknowledged that her performance had in fact declined. She left quietly.

Some months later, the CEO learned that his former employee's mother had died. He further learned from a close colleague that the former COO had been taking care of her sick mother for months before she finally passed away. It occurred to him that it was during that time that he had noticed the slip in performance, and he sadly conceded that had he known what she was going through, he would not have let her go. In fact, he would have wanted to help. What he missed was that in his formal hierarchy, he had created distance with even his close colleagues. He had never asked about the COO's life circumstance, and his working relationships with his employees were so limited that they excluded who they were as people. They never enjoyed the privilege of sharing real-life events, some even of life's difficult times.

Building the bench

Among the most important jobs of the CEO is the recruitment and retention of talented individuals to leadership roles within the organization. This is accomplished mostly through relentless effort and taking interest in individuals throughout the organization. Understanding the importance of "building the bench" is operationalized by maintaining awareness, keeping a written list or mental list of people who demonstrate potential and desire, prompting other senior leaders to maintain awareness and reaching out to individuals directly or through others (HR, direct reports of the CEO) so the "junior" employee is aware that they are "on the radar" for advancement.

The CEO must communicate to other senior leaders that "building the bench" is an important and ongoing effort and is defined as having people ready to take on management and leadership responsibility when an opening occurs. This is a major factor in the organization's overall future success as when someone does leave, there is a short list of potential candidates available to fill a gap in personnel. This allows the organization to maintain momentum by not having to devote precious time to what can be a lengthy process of searching for and recruiting candidates. It is vital that other senior leaders understand that nurturing talent is a key function of their roles as well. The CEO accomplishes this through modeling nurturing behavior, through ongoing inquiry with other senior leaders about individuals in their areas of responsibility, and through making this an area of evaluation in performance reviews of senior leaders.

There are a variety of creative ways for the CEO to demonstrate interest in particular individuals in the organization, though it is mainly just a matter of taking the time to reach out. One of the best ways is to acknowledge some work achievement or milestone with a brief note or email to the individual and a copy of that communication to the person's supervisor (and often that person's direct supervisor). Many organizations have recognition programs that honor individuals for their efforts and compassion, and acknowledgment from the CEO at these moments adds to the power of those awards. Another effective way is to invite an individual to participate in an event such as a training opportunity, a committee, or task force that brings together individuals from across the organization. The main goal is to let the individual know that they have been noticed and that there is organizational interest in facilitating their engagement in the broader workings of the organization. All these activities set the stage for increased connectedness of individuals to each other and to the organization.

Example

A creative idea that turned into a powerful organizational structure is a management training program we named the President's Fellows program. This started with individuals in the organization being nominated by a supervisor for a ten-month training program and then having the individual write a brief biography and answer a series of questions that focused more on career goals and areas of personal growth. These applications are then reviewed by the CEO and a "class" of six or seven people is selected to participate. The selected class is announced to the entire organization. As this is planned as an annual opportunity, individuals who are not selected (often due to class size limitations) are encouraged to re-apply the following year.

The chosen individuals often have little real management experience, so the President's Fellows program is designed to jump start their acquisition of skills and knowledge and provide an in-depth exposure to every part of the organization. In addition to meeting as a group with the CEO every quarter, the class has scheduled meetings with the vice presidents of each major department. Vice presidents are instructed to provide an overview of their department and encourage discussion and questioning. Each department head highlights how their department is essential to the running of the organization. On the Fellows part, there is permission and encouragement to learn as much as possible and to walk away from each meeting with a sense of understanding of each department. In addition to the learning component, there is a requirement that each Fellow identify a problem area within the organization, develop a creative idea designed to improve the situation, and begin a plan for implementing their solution. All projects are reviewed in a meeting with senior leadership at the end of the ten months.

The projects are impressive. Many of the Fellows work in the front lines of the organization and have a perspective on problem areas that may have gone undetected in the past. For instance, one Fellow, coming from the finance department was frustrated that he had to look through numerous reports every day to get an accurate read on the overall census for the organization. For his project, he was able to work across all clinical departments and proposed a single census spreadsheet that pulled an accurate census across all levels of care and all locations. With his knowledge of each department and newly built relationship with the department heads, he was able to implement a new single census report that went into practice almost immediately. It was an impressive undertaking and highly effective in providing critical information.

We found the program so successful that it became an anticipated process throughout the organization. Employees interested in growing in their careers look forward to the application process and once selected are excited about what they will learn and the organization's investment in them. As we anticipated, the President's Fellows program is a highly effective stairway to advancement in the organization often feeding open management positions with newly trained and motivated talent.

Social engagement

Over the years, we have found that it is vitally important to foster relationship building across the organization. We do this in a variety of planned ways, including joint trainings, both in person and via video conferencing, participation in organizational activities such as the DEI (Diversity, Equity, Inclusion) task force, and through less structured social events such as company celebrations and company-sponsored afterwork gatherings. More and more, as we have observed the powerful effects of getting to know one's peers, we have thought of these social events strategically as both the "social glue" and the "social lubricant" that enhances company functioning.

While it is common for organizations to host social events, our conclusion is that these events play an important role and provide benefits to patients in a Behavioral Health System of Care. So often, we have observed staff from different parts of the organization who have collaborated on complex cases via email, text, and medical record meeting each other for the first time in person on one of these occasions. They always come away from the meetings with greater comfort now that they can put a face with a name and have had direct interaction with their colleagues. This accrues to the benefit of patients especially at moments of transition: a referring clinician is much more reassuring to his/her patient when he/she "knows" who is receiving the patient on the other end and the receiving clinician is likely to spend more time and additional consideration to the information that is being shared by the referring clinician. This is how continuity of care is operationalized.

Example

As Walden Behavioral Care started to expand, the CEO noticed signs that communication between programs had become distant and, in some cases, strained. The valued warm hand-off of a case in the acute care hospital to another program in the system, once easily done to a trusted colleague in that program, had shifted. People didn't know one another. In many respects, he reasoned that it was a natural consequence of growth. In the past, there were many opportunities for clinicians to see each other and over time many friendships developed. With those relationships, sending a patient to another site was like sending someone to visit a trusted friend. The patient and the entire system benefited. The problem was that with growth, something we all welcomed, came a physical distance between programs and decreased opportunities for people to get to know each other organically. In some cases, clinicians in more distant programs had never had the opportunity to get to know clinicians in other programs.

The CEO initiated a project in which he challenged the clinician group at the acute care hospital to visit each of the new program sites with the goal of improving communication. Some of the programs were relatively close with travel times under an hour, but others were far away and for the acute care team would require at least half the day. The details of the project were specific. The acute care team would travel to the program site and meet all the clinical staff there. They were to have a meeting in which they would review a case that had gone well, intentionally focusing on successes, the small steps that made the case go well. There was an effort to identify success points that each team would want to continue. Afterward, both teams were to do something fun together. This could be an outside game, lunch, or dinner, or simply going out for drinks. The goal was to have the group get to know each other outside of their work environment.

While some may think such effort and expense is frivolous, the results were tangible. With very little time spent, clinicians in one program got to know each other and that small beginning grew with the day-to-day work of referring patients and phone calls. What was remarkable was the fondness that one team could express to our patients for the receiving team. It was as if a patient was being sent to visit a friend. At the end of each visit, there was a plan developed for the program team that was visited to return the favor and visit the acute care setting.

Chief medical officer (CMO)

Whether the title is CMO, Medical Director, Chief of Psychiatry, or Chief Clinical Officer, the person who is responsible and accountable to the CEO for overseeing the organization's medical and clinical practices and programs is of singular importance in a Behavioral Health System of Care. The CMO is a near co-equal in impact and influence to the CEO. There are a host of important skills and qualities that are important for any medical leader (not discussed here) and several specific qualities and convictions that are critical in a Behavioral Health System of Care setting.

Most importantly, the person in this role must understand that virtually everyone in the organization looks to them and their direct reports on the medical staff (medical doctors, nurse practitioners, clinical psychologists, and other senior clinical staff) as models of relational behavior. *What this means is that the CMO is the chief tone setter for the clinical enterprise of the organization, and they must embrace, in word and deed, a "model of team collaboration."* Professional collaboration within programs and sub-components and across the entire system is, by far, the best approach for supporting the recovery of individuals with moderate to severe psychiatric illness. And it is not easy. In fact, most healthcare in the United States is built firmly on the medical model, a highly hierarchical structure which positions the medical provider as the authority in all matters related to treatment. It is unusual for a system to operate with a spirit of true collaboration, and when it does, it is often to the credit of the CMO. Their conviction, valuing the contributions of all staff, and "way of being" must be present in a Behavioral Health System of Care and should be apparent in the orientation and behavior of the CMO and other senior clinical leaders' behavior in the organization.

In behavioral health, an area of medicine that has become increasingly focused on psychopharmacology, this requires an individual who while versed in the utility of behavioral health medications knows well their limitations. They must be cognizant and valuing of the work with other disciplines in treatments that are not always medical in orientation. A good CMO not only does this partnership comfortably, but they are able to communicate to their medical staff that "this is how we work here; it is our culture."

Second, a strong CMO operates in the spirit of true curiosity. This is a trait that is essential when working with complex patients who have often exhausted conventional medication trials and treatments and perplexed past treaters. Through true curiosity, the CMO invites all to participate. There is no pride in ownership with anyone welcome to contribute their thinking and work toward a solution. Systems that have this part of medical leadership in place are best positioned to create forward movement in care for individuals who otherwise might remain stagnant.

Of course, all senior leaders, including the CMO, are expected to support the mission and values of the organization and operate in synch with the CEO. The CMO, however, has unique influence in messaging the organization about the importance of accepting responsibility *as an organization* for treating difficult patients with sensitivity and to the dignity of the patient and family. The CMO models a treatment style which does not blame either individual patients or individual staff when the desired clinical outcomes are not fully achieved. Setting this standard of acceptance is foundational and has far-reaching implications for patients and staff and, by extension, for the organization and the success of the business.

When it is widely acknowledged that our collective raison d'etre, our reason for existence, is to provide care to complex patients without judgment, the entire organization is enriched. In achieving that, the CMO maintains a conviction of the possibility of recovery despite the difficulties and reality of a patient's current condition. With this, we avoid getting mired in the issue of "what went wrong" or "who messed up" and focus instead on "what can we do now to improve the situation." It might be obvious, but it should be stated that in accepting responsibility for providing this orientation to treatment that "makes a difference," the CMO communicates confidence that the Behavioral Health System of Care has the necessary resources and programs to do the job.

The CMO must be knowledgeable and current with the offerings of each program and instructive and supportive of the system operating smoothly, particularly by helping to define and ease transitions in care when a particular clinical situation or complex patient becomes "stuck." The CMO or designee (depending on the need for a specific expertise) may be called upon to be the final arbiter of a situation where programs and/or clinicians raise serious concerns about an impending discharge or move to another level of care or program. In these situations, it is important for the CMO to be seen as an "honest broker" who has equal regard (i.e. no favoritism) for each of the components of the system.

Chief operating officer (COO)

The COO, sometimes known as the Vice President of Operations or other similar title, is the individual who is accountable to the CEO and responsible for the efficient and effective day-to-day operations of the Behavioral Health System of Care. This is first and foremost a business function, but it often requires extensive knowledge of clinical enterprise and the day-to-day needs of patients and staff.

We have found that having a clinical background can be very helpful for a COO as it brings with the title a sensitivity to the nuances that often accompany behavioral health treatment as well as providing a sense of credibility among behavioral health providers. Whether the individual has a clinical background and training or not, the COO must have a skill set that allows them to effectively manage the operation in a comprehensive manner. They must be decisive, capable of managing multiple tasks with what might appear to be ease, and able to communicate effectively with clinicians who comprise most of the staff in the programs.

Given that behavioral health is often more amorphous than the black and white of many industries, the COO must be able to make quick decisions often without achieving a consensus. In this respect, it can be a lonely job with multiple priorities to manage (often at the same time). Because of this, it is important that the COO be a consistent presence in the organization and have a pulse on the day-to-day operations. Where there is an irregularity or problem, it is their job to quickly assess and implement a remedy with a direct and respectful approach. The COO works closely with the CEO, CMO, and other senior leaders to produce excellent business results while still upholding the central tenets of the organization's mission and vision.

In many respects, the COO is at the "center of the wheel" assisting the CEO and ensuring that other aspects of the business operation (finance, HR, marketing) are also doing what they need to do to achieve expected business outcomes. We think of this often as a provider-customer relationship, with the provider being the many supports in the organization and the customer being the individuals in the organization most directly interfacing with the patient and their family.

When a problem occurs with another department or a delay of some sort, the COO must be able to intervene quickly and pull in whatever resources are needed to resolve the problem. For example, food services seem to be a frequent challenge in many twenty-four-hour care programs. Of course, food is a daily need and it's hard to please everyone. There are specific diets, allergies, and preferences to manage, with a complexity that can grow quickly, especially when someone might miss a meal. So, when there is no vegetarian option on the menu, there must be a quick resolution. If the solution doesn't occur in the food service department, the situation can escalate to the COO who must assess the situation, develop some options (often right on the spot), and direct personnel often from different departments. If the problem turns out to be a larger one which requires a longer-term solution, it may need further review and discussion in a more formal manner. Although many problems may not seem critical to the larger functioning of the organization, the presence and timely response of the COO is critical. Embedded in the responsiveness of the COO are messages to the program staff about how assertively we work to resolve areas of concern for our patients and families and how we work together as a team.

This "team mentality" is central to the work of the COO who will rely on teams to identify and resolve problems throughout the organization. In practice, they will convene many teams of middle managers for varying purposes associated with the operation of programs and departments. In doing this, it is critical for the COO to work in a collegial and complimentary fashion, allowing each employee permission to solve problems themselves in the best interests of patients and when creative solutions are developed for unanticipated events, to participate fully and with enthusiasm.

The COO must work closely with the CMO so that business decisions do not compromise clinical integrity and are made with a full understanding of the needs of the clinical operation. The support of the CMO underscores the importance of a well-run enterprise for stability in patient care and for the longevity of the enterprise. The COO works continually to maintain efficient operations and weighs the needs of the organization in the areas of utilization and resource management, often working through other leaders and assisting with day-to-day problem solving. A strong COO can facilitate innovation that allows the programs to function smoother and expand or improve their services.

It is important for the COO, like the CEO and CMO, to support each component of the system similarly and assist the programs and thus the system to function smoothly by sharing information and moving patients as easily as possible as their needs change. In doing this, they work to create a culture that moves the organization forward and creates a healing environment for patients and families.

Chief nursing officer (CNO)

Almost all Behavioral Health Systems of Care that operate an acute care program or hospital will have a Chief Nursing Officer (CNO) or a Director of Nursing. This is a critical leadership position in part due to the size and scope of the Department and the reality that the number of employees involved can have a decisive impact on the culture of the entire organization. Strong behavioral health systems are known for their nursing department and a good CNO can be the heart and soul of a program. Alternatively, an indifferent one can hobble what otherwise might be a great program into mediocrity

In a Behavioral Health System of Care, the nursing department is generally comprised of nurse leaders, licensed nurses who oversee the day-to-day management of a unit or program, and often a group of paraprofessionals who work under the direction of the nurses to deliver direct care services patients and to maintain program safety. In our systems, we have always sought nurses who specialize in behavioral health who work together with paraprofessionals such as Mental Health Counselors (MHCs). Their importance to the successful running of an acute care setting cannot be overstated.

It is incumbent on the CNO to create a hierarchical structure which delineates lines of accountability and communication and through which all staff members are recruited, hired, and trained. This structure includes nursing supervisors across all shifts, charge nurses who oversee each shift on each floor or program, and staff nurses who can manage the day-to-day nursing tasks of the program. We also endorse an accompanying hierarchy for Mental Health Counselors and have used senior MHCs as mentors for the training and oversite of newer and often younger employees. These combined personnel staff programs operate twenty-four hours a day every day of the year. Given the size of the group and the intensity of the work that a nursing department provides, the department must have a structure that supports communication flow to each level and a rapid response for events that require immediate attention.

As an administrator, the CNO must have what we will broadly describe as professional leadership and "presence." They must exemplify and enforce a high standard of nursing practice and through their presence communicate that high standard as an expectation for each of the employees in the department. As the CNO is often the primary role model for this level of professionalism, it is their "presence" that creates a healthy culture. Simply stated, they must be seen and available to their employees and known as someone who can move with confidence whether that be managing a crisis, organizing a shift with changing or limited resources, and most importantly in modeling how patients and their families will be spoken to, about, and treated.

This sense of presence is not easy to achieve. Certainly, the CNO will need to have a physical presence in the program, something that can be achieved with a flexible work schedule which allows the CNO to show up regularly at off shifts and the ability to develop working relationships with program staff. But the greater sense of presence is in creating a shared group awareness of the standard of care that is set by the CNO, and most importantly, how that is operationalized. A strong nursing program has internalized a sense of how the CNO thinks and how the CNO would want a situation handled. When the program staff achieve an internalized sense of the CNO's presence, they will collectively address problems of challenges in that manner consistent with the CNO's standards even when the CNO is not available.

Last, a CNO must be relentless in pursuing ongoing training and support for program staff. In many of these programs, the individuals hired come with a high level of good will but little training. Most programs will offer some basic orientation in the first few weeks of employment to meet the needs of completing the basic functions of a job. This is the easy part and can be developed and implemented through an orientation program. We have even seen programs in which components of a basic orientation are done either in person or virtually through professional training video. The bigger challenge is in developing the opportunity for ongoing learning which can align with and enhance the employees actual practice experience. Ongoing training can be a powerful means for systematically supporting nurses and MHCs in their work as it not only adds to the clinical sophistication of the program but enhances the direct care staff members job satisfaction in the behavioral health field.

Related, and a critical part of training, is creating a system in which direct care staff have the opportunity for consistent and supportive supervision. This differs from orientation or topic-specific training in that the intent is to allow staff members to express their own concerns in a learning format. It is particularly powerful if the facilitator can link what staff members are seeing and experiencing on a day-to-day basis, and how they feel with how to respond to a patient's need most effectively. This form of supervision is essential after a particularly difficult event or shift and fosters growth in behavioral health work that is essential in maintaining and developing staff members over time.

Chief human resource officer

Most organizations have a Chief Human Resources Officer, sometimes referred to as the Chief People Officer, who is the leader of the Human Resources Department, a group which exclusively focuses on the needs of the employees within the organization. This department is the face of company caring, especially relating to health insurance and special situations that may arise for individual employees. As a system of care is always about the employees, this department is often the unsung hero in terms of developing and maintaining the tone and culture of the organization. To marginalize this function is a strong negative signal to employees and would likely hamper the organization's effort to hire and retain the talent needed to create excellence.

The scope of responsibilities within the Human Resources Department is large and includes everything from payroll systems and personnel policies to assisting employees in their career development through training, tuition assistance, and internal advocacy for equitable pay and benefits. In some organizations, the Human Resource Department has a limited role and can take on the feel of an enforcer of policy and manager of untoward behavior through corrective action plans. But in a strong organization, the Chief Human Resources Office leads a team that is capable of fostering a sense of connection among employees and ultimately a feeling of community.

The Chief Human Resources Officer plays a significant role in setting this tone, often through how employees are thought of and spoken about and ultimately in how they are treated by the organization. Because of this, it is imperative that the Chief Human Resources Officer resonates with the culture set by the senior leadership group. We have always encouraged the Chief Human

Resource Officer to think and work creatively to engage employees, finding a lot of success in enjoyable events that occur outside of the work setting. Efforts directed toward the goal of connecting employees with one another as people, outside of their work roles, is a valuable organizational investment.

References

Berghout, M. A., Fabricotti, I. N., Buljac-Samardzic, M., and Hilders, C. G. J. M. (2017). Medical leaders or masters? - A systemic review of medical leadership in hospital settings. *PLoS ONE*, 12(9), e0184522. http://doi.org/10.1371/journal.pone.0184522.

Cliff, B. (2012). Patient centered care: The role of healthcare leadership. *Journal of Healthcare Management*, 57(6), 381–383.

O'Brien, M. (2008). Leading innovation in a risk-averse healthcare environment: The role of the healthcare CFO is changing. *Healthcare Financial Management*, 62(8), 112+. Gale Academic OneFile, link.gale.com/apps/doc/A192352075/AONE?u=mlin_oweb&sid=googleScholar&xid=f0f978d1

Zimring, C., Augenbroe, G. L., Malone, E. B., and Sandler, B. L. (2008). Implementing healthcare excellence: The vital role of the CEO in evidence-based design. *HERD: Health Environments Research & Design Journal*, 1(3), 7–21.

9

BUSINESS CONSIDERATIONS

Regardless of whether a Behavioral Health System of Care is public or privately funded or both, there are key business considerations that drive development decisions and ongoing management of the System. These considerations and decisions may be quite different depending on the payer, specifically in a public versus private enterprise. For example, managing the interface with payers varies greatly in a publicly funded system where the payer is always some form of government, either at a local, state, or federal level. With government funding comes a detailed and prescribed process for the procurement and payment of any service. These are often time-consuming processes that can present a challenge for any request to modify an existing service.

In the privately funded world, things can be quite different. Though insurance companies can vary greatly in terms of their flexibility, each likely has a detailed process for authorization, payment, and any modification. Unlike public sector payers, there is usually a specific decision maker or group that has the authority to make a change, often in a shortened timeframe. Funding a system of care to meet a need identified by the insurance company or making changes in how services are delivered or priced can occur quickly. And in fairness, there are areas in which the two systems are quite similar. We see this frequently when considering such areas as Human Resources or models of leadership. In this chapter, we consider both privately funded and publicly funded Behavioral Health Systems of Care, where there are major differences and where they overlap.

DOI: 10.4324/9781315177366-10

Relevant history of managed care

Sixty years ago in the United States, private, independent healthcare practitioners were available to all who could afford them. Many medical services were reimbursed through employer-purchased, low-cost, indemnity insurance plans (DeKruif 1943). These plans offered the subscriber a choice of practitioner with little or no regulation of expense or quality. The subscriber was essentially free to choose his or her own community physician, and in turn, the physician was free to choose and deliver a medical intervention or setting that they deemed appropriate based on their professional training. What service was needed was determined exclusively by the treating professional with little or no thought of cost. Medical bills were reimbursed by the insurance company for the service rendered.

For several reasons, including improved and expensive technology, financial incentives, and dramatically increasing utilization, medical care costs skyrocketed through the 1970s and 1980s. Employers, increasingly confronted with growing healthcare benefit costs, asked for and then welcomed the introduction of mechanisms that were designed to contain cost escalation. Managed care organizations were formed and employed techniques designed to manage costs. These included quality management, network management, and utilization management and were without question successful in limiting costs (Broskowski 1991).

Broskowski (1991) illustrates the underlying formula of managed care principles as follows:

Total costs = (unit price) × (units used)

With the goal of containing total costs, some mechanisms are designed to reduce utilization (units used) and some mechanisms developed to reduce cost (unit price). Mechanisms designed to reduce units used include pretreatment authorization, concurrent utilization review, cost sharing and benefit plans designed to provide financial incentives or constraints to receive care from efficient providers. Mechanisms which have been developed to reduce unit price include capitated payments, negotiated payments to preferred providers, fixed payments, claims review, and incentives to cover less expensive but equally effective treatment alternatives. A wide array of managed care technologies has been developed and are reviewed by Mizrahi (1993).

A subset of healthcare, mental healthcare, experienced enormous cost escalation during the 1980s. In fact, mental health service costs rose faster than medical costs (England & Vaccaro 1991). Patrick et al. (1993) provided the first empirical evidence that inpatient psychiatric care of children and adolescents was responsive to reductions in benefit coverage rather than the clinical need of the patient. In their review of Blue Cross/Blue Shield Federal Employees Program in 1978 and 1983, they found it "difficult to avoid concluding that the reduction in benefits and shift in the Federal Employees Program population toward low option coverage converged to produce the decrease in use and that these benefit changes overshadowed national trends favoring increases" (p. 151). Managed care plans and plans that specialized in mental health and substance abuse grew (Coffey et al. 1997). Reports show that by 2001, 169 million people were enrolled in a managed behavioral health plan (Fryer 2002), with managed care initiatives continuing to grow from the private sector into the public sector payers.

Prior to all of this, there would have been no possibility of building a Behavioral Health System of Care in the healthcare marketplace. Funding for the development of "sub-acute" services was driven by managed care companies looking for alternatives to expensive inpatient care and scrutinizing rates of treatment efficacy. It is important to note that early development of hospital alternative programs like partial hospital and day treatment programs took place initially in the public sector as state governments and state agencies looked to reduce the number of patients in state hospitals. Landmark lawsuits in numerous states pushed state agencies to make a concerted effort to move patients to community settings, and most importantly, to find ways to support them once there with deinstitutionalization as the initial impetus to the development of sub-acute programming in the public sector. Programs that were intensive but didn't require being in a hospital were developed on hospital grounds and in many cases utilized staff that had previously worked there. These were in essence, the early models for many of the programs that we rely on today to fill in the "mid-section" of the service continuum.

Publicly funded systems of care

While it is true that many treatment models were first developed in the public sector, in our experience, there are very few true systems of care of the kind that we are describing currently operating there. This is not to say that a Behavioral Health System of Care would not work in the public sector. On the contrary, we believe this model would be an important step forward for the public sector. However, both developing and operating such an integrated system of care in the public sector would be exceedingly difficult due to a myriad of issues.

Probably the chief reason is that in the public sector, reimbursement and contracting are complicated. Reimbursements for medical services are different than that of social services reimbursement with state and local governments subject to regulations that tightly govern procurement. For example, hospital level of care is often covered by the two public insurances, Medicaid and Medicare, but other levels of care are not. For example, many Partial Hospital

Programs and Intensive Outpatient Programs are not covered by Medicare. Funding for these and other levels of care must come from state grants to non-profit vendors. And to complicate matters further, these dollars are often spread around to vendors that are tied to specific populations in a community. This makes it very difficult for a single vendor to line up enough contracts of the types needed to adequately construct an integrated system.

Some public entities attempt to provide the services themselves. This rarely works out well as they are often overwhelmed by demands for service. As "provider of last resort," public hospitals and other public programs are asked to be "all things to all people" and with such a broad scope are hard pressed to execute a focused system of care. Additionally, as public entities, there are numerous pressures from other agencies and constituents to admit patients who are problematic for the community. These requests are many and come from state and local politicians looking to aid their constituents as well as judges and courts who are faced with a range of situations that are better handled by medical and social service providers than correctional facilities. While these pressures may have good intentions at their origin, the inability for programs and systems to manage their boundaries according to their stated healing mission creates an untenable situation. As expectations broaden, the clinical structure is eventually rendered generic, creating a mismatch between client need and services offered. In many cases, the outcome to the system is gridlock that interrupts the normal movement and flow of patients.

Case example

Charles River Health Management (CRHM) worked closely with the Department of Mental Health in Massachusetts (1985–1990) to develop a system of care in a public-private partnership model for adolescents in psychiatric distress. Over a relatively brief span of time, CRHM opened and managed a new inpatient unit in a public funded psychiatric hospital, a free-standing residential program, a crisis respite program, and a home-based family therapy program for adolescents who initially required inpatient treatment. These adolescents came with a wide range of psychiatric diagnoses and with complex family situations. There was general agreement between the agency and the vendor that the "system" would provide stabilization and treatment, starting in the inpatient setting and then continuing at lower levels of care as the adolescents' condition improved. Of particular importance, we agreed, was the focus on working with families and loved ones who could provide community and connection to these kids once discharged from the hospital.

The results were initially quite good. As planned, the programs developed and started serving the patients and families. Many of the hospitalized adolescents stepped down from inpatient care to the residential program or the home-based program, with continuing support from the agency and the programs in the system. As this resource became better known in the community, the number of referrals surged and the pressure to admit directly to all levels of care grew beyond any of the programs' capacity. Gridlock occurred at all levels of care, and this prevented movement of cases through the system. This specifically impacted patients at higher levels of care who were not able to step down to another program and adolescents who relapsed were not able to step up when necessary. Patients languished. Although administrative supports were put into place to ease the congestion with some lessening of the problem, it became clear that political pressure outside of the system, often in the form of a court order, was prioritized over the System's operating principles.

Privately funded systems of care

The private sector picked up what had begun in the public sector and contributed with other models such as residential treatment and intensive outpatient treatment. These models were adapted primarily from the substance abuse field where the "30 day stay" in a "retreat" setting was thought to be the humane and necessary environment and time frame for an individual with substance issues to break the habit, and therefore, the treatment of choice. These services were paid for exclusively through private means by individuals and families and sometimes corporations or unions. Intensive outpatient treatment (IOP) was developed as a means of providing intensive treatment for individuals with substance abuse problems who needed more than weekly outpatient counseling and/or Alcoholics Anonymous (AA) groups. They were developed in such a way as to not disturb areas of functioning, especially the structure of daily employment.

Two major problems: One elegant solution

Our review of private and publicly funded "systems" in behavioral health describes the main problems that impacted, and to some extent, continue to impact these two different worlds. In the private arena, soaring costs led to business strategies and practices targeted to cost containment. In the public sector, the soaring need for treatment and the recognition that large state hospitals were not the answer led to the development of new non-facility-based models of care. Taken together, these pressures have led to the emergence of what we call sub-acute care, the mid-section or mid-range of care comprised of all the services that exist between hospital level of care and simple outpatient care. This also creates the opportunity, certainly for the first time in known history of the field, to align these various models and levels of treatment intensity to provide a continuous treatment experience for patients and a more efficient way for them to move toward health.

Behavioral Health Systems of Care as a business strategy

Behavioral Health Systems of Care are the best way for patients to get care and they are also a sound business strategy for several reasons. We consider this a "happy circumstance:" it is just one of those things in life that happenstance turned out to be good for all parties. Most of this book is about the why and how of Behavioral Health System of Care and its beneficial attributes for patients. But what makes it good business?

One customer, multiple "sales"

There are several things about operating a Behavioral Health System of Care that make it a good business opportunity if done in the right way. First, is that unlike many other behavioral health businesses that provide one level of care (i.e. a hospital or an outpatient practice or a residential program), the patients who utilize any level of care in a Behavioral Health System of Care organically become consumers for other levels of care and other programs. Another way to say this is that when new patients are admitted or "acquired," business parlance indicating a paying customer or sale, they often use more than one service in their treatment episode. This greatly reduces the cost to the business of acquiring new patients. And that's a big issue for these businesses because they must operate at high volume to cover their substantial costs, produce surplus (aka "margin" or "profit") for expansion and continued improvement, and provide a return on investment for private funders. A Behavioral Health System of Care is only viable and will be judged positively as a business if it is operating at a high percentage of its capacity. The primary metric of business success is "productive time," the degree to which Behavioral Health System of Care resources whether they be beds (inpatient, residential), slots (day treatment, partial hospital, intensive outpatient), or clinical hours (outpatient) are being utilized by paying customers.

A related point to the advantage of a Behavioral Health System of Care serving patients at multiple levels of care is the difference this creates from other programs with single or few levels of care. In a Behavioral System of Care, there are multiple levels through which to move patients. This is especially true when one has an inpatient unit as a key component to the system. Here, the inpatient unit serves as an anchor for the entire system, receives and sends referrals to other programs, and diminishes the risk of losing its patients to another program when they require "step up" or intensification of services.

This occurs with great frequency when programs are serving individuals with complex psychiatric illnesses. We know that recovery from these disorders is not linear, and it is not uncommon for a patient who is in treatment to have a temporary reversal of progress and need the safety and security of residential or inpatient care. When a program or service does not have that next, needed intensive program, the patient is often referred out, likely to another program or system and frequently does not return. Having a hospital level of care as part of the Behavioral Health System of Care provides the ultimate in clinical backup and support. And importantly, it greatly decreases the possibility that a patient will be referred out of the system.

Average daily census (ADC), the holy grail of behavioral health programs and businesses

Any discussion about the business of mental health must appreciate the centrality of the issue of census. Indeed, for some, this is the only issue that they deem important. Hopefully, this book challenges that tenet, but we do agree that census and especially the lack of census or underutilization of program capacity is a first-level concern.

The word "census" is used in behavioral health as shorthand to refer to the concept of volume, specifically patient volume, the number of patients receiving services on any given day or period of time. It originates most likely from the practice of taking the count of patients in a hospital (i.e. "taking the census") at midnight which is the methodology prescribed by the Centers for Medicare Services (CMS) for billing and reimbursement. Any patient "on the census" at midnight is billable, and this is the beginning of the chain of operational procedures that eventually result in the organization receiving reimbursement for the services it provides. Average daily census ADC is the key metric that behavioral health administrators, CEOs, CFOs, program directors, etc. use to monitor service volume and, critically, the amount of revenue that will result from their program operations once the revenue cycle (billing and collections) is complete. Anyone operating a mental health facility, program, or service is intimately knowledgeable about census and checks it frequently, especially when the census expectations are not being met.

Behavioral health programs must function at high volume to be successful and stable. This may seem obvious and no different than many other healthcare services or other types of businesses that depend on high customer use and flow, but reimbursement for mental health services has traditionally been low when compared to other medical specialties. While this problem is beginning to get addressed, most payers, including the major government payers, Medicare and Medicaid, originally developed their systems using some rather archaic formulas that determine reimbursement rates. This has disadvantaged mental health services compared to most other areas of healthcare (and commercial insurers followed their lead) and has completely left some licensed clinicians out of the system entirely. Reimbursement for mental health services has also been subject to a high default rate due to difficulties of the population of users in getting and maintaining insurance coverage, meeting expectations for payment of deductibles and services not covered and qualifying or obtaining prior authorization for services as required by managed care organizations.

The major point here is that reimbursement for mental health services is often difficult to capture, and thus, there is little room for error when it comes to operating these services. Utilization rates of at least 75% (average daily census divided by total capacity) are required to achieve sustainability assuming that costs are in line with budget and there is limited expectation of surplus or margin from the program or service. This is particularly true for services that have very high fixed costs such as inpatient services which require twenty-four-hour staffing with nursing and physicians and have high occupancy (building, food, supplies, pharmaceuticals) costs. Many of these facility-based services barely cover their costs at 75% utilization; programs that thrive typically function in the high eighty percentile and above.

Again, much of what we have said in this section may be obvious, but it's less well recognized or discussed that, in our observation, staff are "happier" and programs function much better when they are busy. It seems that predictability is extremely important to staff assuming there are reasonable resources to meet the demand of the consumers/patients that they are serving.

In addition, high census implies a general recognition that the service is important, imparts a sense of stability, and sharpens the clinical focus; in other words, "we're good, we have an important job to do, and we cannot mess around." Also important to this sense of well-being is the feedback that staff get from the administration. When the program is "humming," the administrators and managers are expressing or exuding positiveness, eager to be identified as leaders of the service and, perhaps, even talking about expansion. This creates a cycle of positive regard and heightened investment in the work that is taking place. In a program that is underperforming and not meeting its census expectations, the managers are grim, thinking and talking about how to cut costs, and looking for reasons why the program is failing. Under these conditions, no one feels good and bad things tend to happen, including the loss of talented staff.

Similarly, when census is high, even important treatment and environmental issues and problems are "challenges" or overlooked altogether; when census is low, minor issues receive more than necessary focus and staff tend to complain and bicker with each other.

Given that high census helps to create a positive work environment and positive momentum, everything within reason should be done to ensure a continuous flow of patients to fill the program capacity. There are important implications here for operations and contracting.

Operational issues that often reduce overall volume are found in admission and discharge procedures that are overly complicated. These processes should be reviewed periodically to see if there are ways to streamline and quicken the pace. In relation to contracting, the primary issue is establishing working relationships with key individuals on the payer side and advocating for initial contracts and contractual rate increases over time. In our experience, there is a benefit to accepting less than optimal rates for services to initiate a source of patient flow. Of course, there are limits as to how low a program or service can go in reimbursement for a service. This requires a detailed cost/benefit analysis, but, in our experience, we have preferred to accept lower rates initially so that we can demonstrate the importance and quality of the services provided and build trust and reliance on our service within the payer organization. Having internal (within the payer organization) "champions" of the work we do then allows us to renegotiate the rates of reimbursement.

Interfacing with insurance companies

In our experience, the interface between a Behavioral Health System of Care and insurance companies or managed care organizations, once established, is less conflictual and more efficient than for single level of care programs. In essence, the logic that managed care companies employ is the same logic that operates within a system of care. Both share the compelling internal logic of providing a range of services that fit together and are specifically designed to support recovery from beginning to end for a particular patient population.

Payors understandably want to spend their care dollars wisely and expect that wherever care is provided, it is essential and that there is ample expertise to provide a high-quality experience for a patient. They also want to avoid the redundancy that occurs throughout much of healthcare in which each admission is a re-start of often repeated past efforts. A Behavioral Health System of Care is built around the idea that individuals may require multiple treatment episodes and provides focused treatment in each setting with professionals who are deep in experience in working with a specific patient population. This allows the Behavioral Health System of Care to have a high degree of credibility with payers, even, at times, being sought after as "the expert" in a clinical area.

Other attractive features of a Behavioral Health System of Care to a payer include the commitment to continuity of care and the built-in structure that makes accessing each level of care relatively seamless. As large insurance companies have employed managed care strategies to create an "oversight" of the healthcare experience, Behavioral Health Systems of Care are structured to have oversight of the patient's treatment course and to see that treatment continues to progress on all identified issues as the patient moves through different programs. There is a far reduced need for the insurance company or payor to be the "glue" or the consistent thread that holds the treatment together. The Behavioral Health System of Care is designed to do that naturally.

Managing managed care through the utilization review process

Collaborating with key payers is essential to the survival and growth of a Behavioral Health System of Care and most align well as a good business partner model. This usually gets played out in the "utilization review" process through which insurance companies monitor key access, performance, and cost indicators. As managed care entities focus on reducing rising healthcare costs, some of the primary drivers of those costs are an overreliance on costly services such as the use of emergency rooms (especially for non-emergent issues) and the expansion and reliance on behavioral health inpatient and residential settings.

Early interventions to contain costs in behavioral health targeted length of stay in these settings with huge effect. As funding constricted, many inpatient units closed and those that remained open found themselves in a new world. Lengths of stay were trimmed to six to ten days when previously three to five times that was the norm. These interventions worked so well that insurance companies found themselves in a position of scarcity of beds and programs to serve their members, so the constraints had to be eased over time. There have also been numerous judgments against managed care companies and insurers for onerous practices and not providing what contractually they have agreed to in their plan documents.

Fast forward twenty years and today we have a less combative situation with managed care companies though they are still trying to keep people out of hospitals and limit the length of stay. Now more than ever, companies are contracting with lower levels of care and encouraging providers to circumvent acute levels of care and admit directly to community-based programs. And patients in acute settings are moved as quickly as possible, sometimes quicker than the clinical teams would prefer.

A Behavioral Health System of Care is less "at the mercy" of managed care's changing Utilization Review practices than single level of care programs or less structured systems. The reasons for this are straightforward: managed care reviewers often begin from a stance of skepticism about the placement of patients in higher levels of care, especially when the entity seeking approval has an ownership interest in that level of care. Understandably, it is perceived as self-serving. In practice, every case that a provider presents to the managed care company for payment is clouded in the perceived self-interest of the provider. In a Behavioral Health System of Care, the incentives are different. There is really no preference to the system as to where the patient is treated; it all depends on what the patient needs at any given time. This orientation to admitting and quickly moving to a less restrictive program is entirely consistent with the stated intention of utilization review.

Example

Things were getting so bad between the medical staff at Walden Behavioral Care and the Utilization Review function at a large national insurer that the Chief Medical Officer decided to step in and handle case reviews himself, thinking that the reports he was receiving had to be grossly exaggerated. His experience was so upsetting after just a few reviews that he came to the CEO and senior leadership group to propose that we stop doing business and forfeit this national account. He reported that not only were the reviewers extremely difficult to reach, but when they finally did appear for the scheduled time, they were demeaning and discourteous, sometimes to the point of insulting. Additionally, the reviews of patients with rather severe disease were rushed and resulted almost always in a denial of the recommended care plan. Something had to be done.

As we thought about what to do, it occurred to us that the reviewers on the other end of the phone while properly credentialed had very little experience with the patient population that we were treating. We reasoned that a better understanding of these patients, our treatment program, and the expertise of our staff might serve to improve the level of the dialog; we had nothing to lose by trying this approach first. This was accomplished by a series of calls to the responsible executives at the insurance company during which we spoke candidly about the current situation and offered a possible solution, namely that representatives of the organization come for a site visit or at least an "electronic" visit, have a direct experience of our clinical program, and attend a brief training session.

This offer was well received, the visit and subsequent training sessions and discussions were held, and the situation improved dramatically. What had been a most difficult and draining experience for our staff became a much more collegial exchange; we were also then asked to provide third-party consultations on clinical situations in other facilities. Indeed, this approach led to a more general effect with our facility becoming a "Center of Excellence" within that insurers network and this, in turn, improved contracting and other administrative interactions as well.

In our experience, when there is a disagreement between the managed care reviewer and a Behavioral Health System of Care clinical evaluator as to where the patient should begin a course of treatment or when they should move to the next level of care, the evaluator can always make the decision to admit to the level of care preferred by the managed care reviewer. We would do this routinely with the proviso that this admission is a "trial" to see if that proposed level of care is sufficient. If it is, fine; we are all to the good. But if it is not, the patient can be easily moved to the correct level of care needed for their current condition.

This is not to say that the Behavioral Health System of Care evaluator or clinician should abdicate responsibility for advocating for the patient to receive the most appropriate care for their condition at that point in time. But it does allow the patient to begin or continue receiving services without interruption during what can become a prolonged negotiation. Our only caveat to this approach is patient safety. If there is a serious question about self-harm or harm to others, there is little room for negotiation around where the patient should be treated.

Using data to inform practice

One of the greatest contributions managed care companies have made to the behavioral health field are sophisticated utilization management information systems. As part of their portfolio, each insurance company has a data system built into proprietary software that allows the capture of critical data points in a patient's treatment experience. Ultimately, all of these are used to make inferences into provider performance which impacts contracting and most importantly, rates.

In many cases, insurance companies today utilize provider profiles for all levels of care they contract for, from complex and expensive services such as an inpatient hospital, to as small as the treatment performance of an individual outpatient clinician. And, in an enhancement to the field, it is common to see individual performances compared against a larger cohort, often a network of like providers. This allows the insurance company to view performance broadly and to manage provider organizations as well as individual providers with corrections to pull more toward the network norm.

This is especially powerful given the sea change it has caused for behavioral health providers, many of whom loathe data and would rebel against the notion of being compared against peers for their performance. Of course, the debate is not over, but in many respects, the battle has already been won. There is no doubt that performance measurement will be a mainstay of practitioners and behavioral health organizations in the future. This presents some opportunities for a Behavioral Health System of Care. We have always believed that we want to be as current in our data collection as any payer we are working with. We have used our Utilization Team to collect and manage data and work to have key indicators available to our managers and directly to our staff, ideally before any discussion begins with a payer. We believe that performance information is essential in a system of care and that the transparency of data provides needed feedback to our staff about how the system is working.

We recommend creating the capacity to capture and track data in any Behavioral Health System of Care. It would be a mistake to allow a payer to define what is happening in your system through the trends identified in their data. And it isn't complicated. Most measures used by payer groups can be found in relatively simple descriptive statistics and without the use of expensive data systems. It is well worth tracking length of stay (both by program and the longer view of a treatment episode) across levels of care. Additionally, critical incidents, re-admission rates, and some specific outcome measures for the illnesses the system is designed to treat. Since all payers can only track data for their members, it is a good idea to be able to view your data by specific payers against all patients in the system. We are learning that in addition to diagnostic presentation, there are distinguishing characteristics for populations covered by certain payers (e.g.public versus private insurances).

The ability of a Behavioral Health System of Care to capture critical data points and to create a picture of the treatment experience of the patients through that data creates an enormous advantage when working with a payer. It is a powerful addition to any discussion when the Behavioral Health System of Care can address a question with data and with an interpretation of that experience through their own lens.

Case example

We meet quarterly with our larger payers and this quarter's meeting began with an overview of a profile report that the managed care company had just developed. It was sophisticated and captured performance data that fed into three important areas: access, cost, and quality. There was no argument that what they were interested in tracking was important in a patient's healthcare experience, though we came to find out that all indicators were not equally weighted. Of critical performance to the managed care company were the indicators related directly to cost, and for this, they looked specifically at length of stay and re-admission rates.

Of note, they had developed the capacity to compare our length of stay and re-admission rates from our hospital against the hundred plus hospitals in their network. And with that, they had created a statistical benchmark, really the average length of stay and expected re-admission rate of their combined network, against which they expected all providers to orient. The message was clear, stay above the mean, and we're good with you. But if you fall below, we have a problem and implied in that message was that they would use whatever means at their disposal to get the errant provider to the mean. It was serious business as it was clear that performance in these indicators would be a factor in the volume of cases, they directed to us as well as any future rate discussions.

We listened thoughtfully to their presentation and interpretation of what their data told them about our system. All seemed well until they got to the critical cost variables: length of stay and re-admission rates. They were perplexed as to why our length of stay was low, but our re-admission rate was seemingly higher than the norm they had established for their network. Fortunately, our Director of Utilization Review was well versed in the data her department collected and used this knowledge to help the insurer understand that what they perceived as an anomaly was actually an expected outcome for our system. She attributed the low length of stay to the flow of the system and our ability to move people quickly out of acute settings and into the community. And in terms of re-admission rate, we discussed using our System to rapidly move someone (briefly) back into the acute care setting when needed.

This led to a useful discussion on how our system is designed to work and ideas about how to better manage outlier cases. She spoke to how we use our continuum of services to move patients through levels of care and that, in a number of cases, we anticipate both forward and backward movement. She reminded them that we did not see stepping someone up to a more acute level of care as a treatment failure, rather as an indicator that the system is responding efficiently to a changing need. And when this does occur, our efforts are focused on getting the person back into the community as quickly as possible. This too was supported in lower lengths of stay.

References

Broskowski, A. (1991). Current mental health care environments: Why managed care is necessary. *Professional Psychology: Research and Practice*, 22(1), 6–14.

Coffey, R. M., Mark, T., King, E., Harwood, H., McKusick, D., Genuardi, J., Dilonardo, J., and Buck, J. A. (1997). *National estimates of expenditures for mental health and substance abuse treatment* (SAMHSA Publication No. SMA-00-3499). Rockville, MD: Center for Substance Abuse Treatment and Center for Mental Health Services, Substance Abuse and Mental Health Services Administration.

DeKruif, P. (1943). *Kaiser wakes the doctors*. New York: Harcourt, Brace and Company.

England, M. J., and Vaccaro, V. A. (1991). New systems to manage mental health care. *Health Affairs*, 10(4), 129–137.

Fryer, F. J. (2002). Managing to get by? MBHOs' future hopes tied to new markets, particularly on private side. (Cover Story) *Behavioral Healthcare Tomorrow*, 11(3), pp. 15. Gale OneFile: Health and Medicine, link.gale.com/apps/doc/A90683312/HRCA?u=mlin_m_bostcoll&sid=bookmark-HRCA&xid=4b53600c. Accessed 26 Aug. 2024.

Mizrahi, T. (1993). Managed care and managed competition: A primer for social work. *Health and Social Work*, 18, 86–91.

Patrick, C., Padgett, D. K., Burns, B. J., Schleslinger, H. J., and Cohen, J. (1993). Use of inpatient services by a national population: Do benefits make a difference? *Journal of the American Academy of Child and Adolescent Psychiatry*, 32, 144–152.

10

ANTICIPATING THE FUTURE

A piece of advice we often give newer clinicians is to avoid predicting the future. We see it as a bit of a behavioral health trap, perhaps forced on us by a public that tends to believe that not only can a therapist read a person's mind, but that somehow a therapist can tell what the future holds. We can't. And the same is true with trying to predict what may likely happen in behavioral health, especially when professions and services are as dynamic as they are at present. But if we take a few learnings from our past and look at the direction we're moving in, there are clear signals of significant changes ahead.

Looking back no one could have anticipated the rapid, even explosive growth of healthcare in the United States over the past decades. What began as soothsayers, sellers of potions and shamans just about a hundred years ago today holds the collective hope of our population for a long life of health and vitality. At the turn of the nineteenth century, medicine was essentially medieval times. Self-proclaimed healers promoted elixirs and magical treatments for almost every malady. Most were woefully ineffective, and medicine had no real basis in science. Things changed in the 1920s with the discovery of Penicillin which became widespread as an effective treatment for infection in the 1940s. The science of modern medicine grew as an effective means to treat illness and so did the public's interest and in turn dollars to pay for basic healthcare. Hospitals proliferated across the country and rudimentary health insurances were developed to pay for them. In the 1960s, Medicare and Medicaid were signed into federal law and eventually become two of today's dominant payers for healthcare. And as part of that, by the 1970s, the fee for service reimbursement system emerged as the primary structure through which medical and behavioral health services

DOI: 10.4324/9781315177366-11

were reimbursed. To this day, the fee for service system remains the dominant structure for reimbursement.

Despite the speed and excitement of medical growth and treatment, behavioral health did not keep up. Providers of care languished with determining what were or were not mental illnesses and ineffective treatments emerged. Many individuals were confined to hospitals. We were limited in our basic understanding of mental illness and operated with a lack of clarity in definitions. Treatments were seemingly anecdotal and with little basis in science, and outcomes were predictably poor. Some were inhumane. Those with mental illness and their families often endured prolonged periods of distress and nationally a stigma against those with mental illnesses became part of our culture and behavioral health landscape.

Today, we have a healthcare industry that has grown into one of the greatest drivers of our national economy and is growing now even faster as the percentage of Americans with health insurance increases through the Affordable Care Act. Behavioral health too is starting to catch up. What started as directionless and with relatively low expectations has grown to the point where the public has a strong belief in the possibility of effective treatment. With each new discovery, our expectations grow even higher.

We have a tremendous amount to figure out to get to the point where we have high-quality behavioral healthcare for all Americans. Although seemingly poised on the precipice of greatness, we are and will continue to experience enormous dips and valleys on our way there. While we can't accurately predict what each hill and valley will be, we believe we can with a degree of certainty identify the battles that must be fought in the necessary evolution of our healthcare system and the critical role that, we hope, systems of care will play in it.

Using the metaphor of a three-legged stool, the behavioral healthcare system has the critical components of access, quality, and cost. The stool works not only because all three legs are needed for it to stand up and work as a stool, but as importantly, because each leg must equally share the total weight of the person sitting on it. It won't work as a stool if one leg is dominant and the other two are weaker. Each area (access, cost, and quality) will have to change in significant ways to fulfill the vision of high-quality, effective, and efficient behavioral health for all.

We first anticipate the continued expansion and growth of systems of care and think that these will develop not as large national systems that dominate the healthcare market but rather as regional systems of care. We reason that people like their "home teams" just like with sports, and in many respects, the same applies to healthcare; we enjoy the concept of choice in providers and draw comfort from a more local feel. Many of these regional systems will integrate behavioral health into a larger medical host system, a significant improvement from how most work today.

However, not all systems will be integrated. We also expect that there will be some large regional behavioral health systems with each made up of smaller behavioral health clusters. Each cluster will specialize in a specific grouping of disorders with providers who work in them trained in treatments specifically designed for the disorders that the system is treating. Gone will be the days when most behavioral health providers are generalists. Specialization in behavioral health will be delivered through systems of care varying according to disorder with treatments based on evidence of effectiveness.

Importantly, we also expect that current annual increases in cost that burden healthcare overall are not sustainable and there will be pressure on healthcare providers to be more focused on outcomes rather than volume of services. One possibility is that payment systems will also be integrated into each large health system. This will mean that each system will essentially be self-insured and will pay itself for services rendered. Larger systems of care will in essence become both the provider and payer of services and the onus will be on each system to develop strong controls to contain costs and to make sure patients are moving appropriately through the levels of care.

Along with large regional systems, there are two factors that dominate healthcare today that we expect will also change. The first is how we broadly define healthcare and by relation how we define the subset that is behavioral healthcare. This gets played out in accessing services as every insurance plan is free to determine what they cover and what they see as "medically necessary" and through that which medically necessary treatments will be paid for. It all varies by payer, and lacking a uniform definition of health care, we find ourselves spending too much time and expense on what is often a poor attempt to match or deny someone's specific need with an existing service and treatment.

Additionally, it is reasonable to expect that as medical research accelerates, it will impact this decision-making. New advances will emerge to assist in the identification of some mental illnesses through genetic markers and in turn the use of genetic information to guide effective treatments. We look forward to the time when disorders that have devastated lives today will become objectively identifiable and with that a course of treatments that will be safe and effective.

The second factor is how services are paid for. Most of the healthcare system uses some version of the fee for service payment system, an old concept in which every service or procedure has a privately negotiated rate that is paid out each time the service is provided. It works well if you're paying someone to cut your lawn or purchasing a pair of pants, but it doesn't make much sense for healthcare. The big problem with the fee for service payment method is that there is a clear incentive on the part of service providers to provide more services. In fact, the more services one can provide the more lucrative their work becomes. A provider makes money only by providing services or procedures to as many people as possible. There is no incentive for a provider to choose a less expensive and still clinically appropriate treatment nor any incentive for any preventative care.

We must create structures within each system of care that financially reward the utilization of less costly treatment and the provision of preventative services. This is where systems of care really have a big opportunity. Unlike a provider's incentive in the fee for service payment system, a system of care has no ingrained incentive to repeatedly provide services. A system's incentive is designed to utilize levels of care to match the clinical need for the patient at any given time rather than repeating expensive treatment services. As the system uses movement to less expensive levels of care to integrate into the community, attention is given to maintaining the flow in a system of care. Payment structures can become more specific to the patient, as in a case rate per patient served, or to movement of the patient through the system rather than the cost of each discrete service.

Given the potential for positive developments in a system of care, there are also some risks, and it is important to highlight them. One risk that seems to be in a state of flux today is the "connection" or interrelatedness of the behavioral health workforce. This refers to the interrelationships that develop among clinicians in behavioral health that are necessary to sustain clinicians in their work. Most people in the field will share a perception that working in behavioral health is different than working in any other setting. Perhaps it is the deeply personal nature of the work in which each clinicians must repeatedly invest themselves in numerous patient relationships and emotionally allow themselves to understand the experience of the patient. Such investment is difficult and over time takes an emotional toll. Colleagues and the relationships that develop by working together are the critical factor that keep people in the field.

We have found that this interrelatedness of the behavioral health workforce is essential and develops through day-to-day connections in the workplace. We are concerned that several developments can erode this connection and, in many cases, create environments in which these connections are not recognized as valuable. We see this risk from the business side with the rapid growth of behavioral health services which often values expansion over investing in the resources needed to create and nourish a supportive culture. While there is a cost to facilitating the development of this culture, decisions not to invest directly into a workforce lead to a loss of connection, disengagement from the work, and poorer outcomes.

Closely related to this is the rise in the use of virtual platforms and the increasing opportunities for clinicians to work from home. While many relish the opportunity to avoid a long commute or the challenge of weather, the result is often that clinicians are seeing patients in relative isolation and rarely have the opportunity for impromptu or formal connections with colleagues. This began during the pandemic with a dramatic shift in the provision and funding of virtual treatments in behavioral health. For over two years, it was the dominant means of providing outpatient care at a time when behavioral health needs were growing and access severely challenged. In many respects, virtual treatment options saved the day. Now, post pandemic, it seems clear that virtual platforms are here to stay as many practitioners continue to work from home.

However, there is a risk. While there is no doubt that going forward these platforms create an opportunity to reach certain populations that might otherwise go underserved (i.e. homebound elders, individuals living in remote locations), it would be a mistake to believe that virtual services are a replacement for meeting with a patient and their family face to face. As clinicians leave behavioral health settings for the convenience of working at home in a virtual-only capacity, we worry about the loss of connection with colleagues both through impromptu and formal meetings.

We are reminded that we have erred in our past by building services that were designed more for the convenience of providers than the needs of patients and families. In behavioral health, the cure or progress comes through a healing relationship, and that there is a qualitative difference between a virtual relationship and one formed in person. We expect this to be especially true for certain populations, like children, where interacting with someone on a screen makes little sense. Similarly, there are some modalities, such as group programming which seem to translate poorly to a screen.

This isn't to say that virtual service provision should go away. On the contrary, it does provide a valuable service to some and will most certainly remain a part of the behavioral health landscape. But it is important to monitor and research the use of virtual platforms for treatment effectiveness. In the meantime, we encourage the development of hybrid models which include a mixture of face-to-face and virtual platforms as an option for building both a treatment relationship and improving access.

We have a similar caution with the introduction of artificial intelligence in recent years. There are lots of predictions about AI growth and sometimes worrisome tales of how it will impact almost all healthcare fields, including behavioral health. At present, there are models available that when prompted can provide a computer-generated response that is designed to read as if a therapist had written it. It can be adjusted to personality type and problem area and is informed by a wealth of digitalized behavioral health knowledge. No one really knows how quickly AI will become a significant part of the behavioral health landscape or the degree to which those seeking behavioral health will find it an effective intervention. However, AI does present some important advantages in terms of access and cost. And of course, some risks.

On the plus side, accessing an AI service will be easy and could be available to anyone at any point in a day or night, even during a time of crisis, with relatively low cost. While our concerns for AI are like those of virtual services in that the relationship is not a human connection, for an emerging generation of Americans, this may be a workable solution. Most Americans readily turn to the internet for answers to almost anything and certainly use it to get information and even support about significant life problems. It is likely that for many, the availability of behavioral health through AI will be highly appealing. There will be no appointments to keep nor concerns of matching with the "right" therapist. And if it isn't working in the manner one wants, with a click, there will be many other options to choose from.

What we really don't know is whether AI interventions in behavioral health will be effective in creating behavioral change. From our perspective as senior therapists, we see much of the art of therapy is not in providing the "right" answer or solution to an individual. In fact, therapists who approach treatment in such a way may miss one of the most important considerations in therapy: that being the possibility that most people intuitively know what to do to solve a problem. They are not looking for someone to tell them what to do. What they struggle with is why they can't do what they know they must do. Figuring that out is a longer, more introspective journey of discovery and often happens through the nuances of a relationship with a good therapist. These nuances, to be more specific, are the silent pauses in a discussion, the moments of recognizing and sitting with a difficult emotion, and often in the struggle to put it into words when a strong feeling is emerging. That is the distinctly human part of therapy and likely not something that can be programmed into AI.

That being said, we do believe that AI will have a place in behavioral health in the future and specifically a role in systems of care. AI can play a significant role in connecting people with similar areas of struggle with one another and could potentially bring them together as both an educator, by sharing current information in the field, and as a facilitator in discussion. We can imagine a time when levels of care will be complemented by AI perhaps as a means for providing support around the clock, particularly during periods of transition and as a powerful resource that can assist people in maintaining the gains they have made from treatment.

In closing

At the end of the day, systems of care are not buildings, equipment, or procedures. They are people who commit to working together to treat a set of distinct illnesses in concert. After decades working in behavioral health, we have experienced both the power of a system of care and the painstaking challenges they present to make them true places of healing and we are convinced that a system of care is the best means for treating a challenging set of disorders in the most humane way. About this we are passionate.

In these chapters, we have described the philosophy, culture, and components that we believe create the structure for a system of care to work well and to provide a realistic treatment course, but success is always about the people. The best systems have exceptional leadership, hire the right people, provide specific diagnostic-related training, and build a supportive culture that retains talent over time. It is our hope that our belief and thinking about a system of care will influence the future of behavioral health. This roadmap for building such a system is our legacy.

INDEX

Note: Figures are indicated by the page number followed by "*f*" and the figure number e.g., *15f1.2* refers to figure 1.2 on page 15.